Assessing and Treating
Late-Life Depression

Assessing and Treating

Late-Life Depression

A Casebook and Resource Guide

MICHELE J. KAREL,
SUZANN OGLAND-HAND AND
MARGARET GATZ,
WITH JÜRGEN UNÜTZER

BASIC BOOKS
Basic Books
A Member of the Perseus Books Group

Published by Basic Books,
A Member of the Perseus Books Group

Designed by Deborah Gayle

Karel, Michele J.
Assessing and treating late-life depression : a casebook and resource guide / Michele J. Karel, Suzann Ogland-Hand, and Margaret Gatz ; with Jürgen Unützer.
p. cm.
Includes bibliographical references and index.
ISBN-10 0–465–09543–7
ISBN-13 978-0–465–09543–8
1. Depression in old age. I. Ogland-Hand, Suzann. II. Gatz, Margaret. III. Unützer, Jürgen.

RC537.5 .K37 2002
618.97'68527–dc21

2001043855

To my parents:
Irving and Phyllis Karel

–MJK

To my parents:
M. Susan Ogland and the late Ervin N. Ogland

–SOH

Contents

Preface

We wrote this book because we love working with older adults and we want to convey the importance and reward of helping individuals who suffer from late-life depression find pleasure, acceptance, or reduced suffering. The strength and perspective that many older adults possess are often inspiring, as is the commitment many families bring to caring for frail elders. Many people who experience depression in late life do not get treatment although we know–from the research literature and our clinical experience–they can benefit from psychotherapy, antidepressant medication, care management, or a combination of these approaches. We hope this book will help you to appreciate the need and various approaches for, as well as the professional reward of, recognizing and treating depression in older adults.

Let us mention our professional backgrounds. The three primary authors (MK, SOH, MG) are clinical geropsychologists: we are psychologists who specialize in the assessment and treatment of, and methods of research for studying, mental health issues in late life. As such, we are committed to a biopsychosocial conceptual framework and to interprofessional collaboration in geriatric care. While the book is clearly influenced by our backgrounds in clinical psychology–for example, most of the case studies include a psychotherapy component of care–we hope that the material we discuss will appeal to a broad range of professionals who work with depressed elders. Primary care, community-based, and specialty mental health providers are all critical points of contact for recognizing, referring, and/or treating geriatric depression.

This book would not have been possible without the courageous older adults who allowed us to be part of their lives for a brief time. We want to thank our clients, whose willingness to work with us has enriched our lives. And, while no one case presented herein is entirely true (i.e., all confidentiality has been maintained), the compilation and integration of their stories will hopefully serve to help other elders receive effective care for depression.

We also wish to acknowledge the contribution of several individuals in particular who helped us to make this book a reality. First, thanks to Jürgen Unützer, geriatric psychiatrist, for consulting with us: for writing the appendix on medications, drafting the chronic pain case study, and reviewing the entire manuscript with care and constructive feedback. Thanks to Cindy Hyden, our editor, who went "above and beyond" in so many ways; her ability to envision the big picture, as well as attend to fine details, was very, very helpful.

Michael Smyer provided the initial impetus for getting this project off the ground and for this we thank him. The Robert Ellis Simon Foundation provided early support. We appreciate Brendan Lynch's excellent research assistance, and Margaret Staudt's practical, easy-to-understand answers to medical questions. Thanks to Greg Hinrichsen, Millie Astin, and Wayne Katon for their reviews and helpful comments on the complicated grief and PTSD chapters and the antidepressant medication appendix, respectively. Thanks to Jennifer Moye, Scott Roberts, and Deborah McKee for reading and providing valuable comments on specific sections of the manuscript.

Finally, we are truly grateful to our families and friends –with special thanks to Mark, Jonathan, and Callie Ogland-Hand, and Mark Green–for encouraging our commitment to this project and cheering us on despite the time it took from usual weekend activities!

PART ONE

Background

CHAPTER ONE

Setting the Stage

> Marie, an attractive and outgoing woman of 75, could not believe how her life had changed over the past ten years. When her husband was diagnosed with lung cancer, she retired from part-time work at the art museum gift shop; he died two years later. At first she found comfort in her church and companionship with several women friends. But with developing complications from her diabetes, including peripheral neuropathy and vision changes, she was no longer feeling confident to drive. The small house she had lived in for forty-three years was several miles from town, too far to walk for church, shopping, or other errands. She dearly missed her best friend Betty, who had moved to a distant nursing home after her stroke. Marie's three children had settled out-of-state years earlier and, although one daughter was hinting that Marie move out to be with them, she could not imagine giving up her home and community.
>
> Everything had become an effort; she was walking less and cooking less and grew reluctant to ask church members for rides. She had little patience for trying to read and couldn't concentrate; with increasingly poor sleep at night, she felt tired all the time. When she shared her troubles with her doctor, he prescribed an antidepressant medication. But her fixed income barely covered the cost of it in addition to her other medications. Marie felt stuck.

Older adults who become depressed often have a number of interacting problems, as well as personal resources upon which to draw. Marie's challenges include coping with grief, physical discomfort, vision loss, decreased independence, distant social supports (children), limited access to affordable medical care, and tough decisions (like where to live). Her strengths include a long history of positive coping, strong relationships, and spiritual commitment. Helping clients like Marie means appreciating this complexity and being open to a range of interventions that can decrease depression and improve quality of life.

Who Is an "Older Adult"?

The definition of "old" seems to get older as we do. As people are commonly living well into their eighties and nineties, we apply the word at later and later ages. Even if we identify 65 as roughly the beginning of "late life," in keeping with the start of social benefit programs, we recognize that, on average, the experiences of the "young-old" differ greatly from those of the "old-old." The meaning of an individual's age, particularly as relevant to understanding and treating depression, depends on the interaction of developmental, historical, and societal factors (Knight and McCallum, 1998).

People who have lived for 75 years, like Marie, have that many years of experience informing who they are and how they have coped with life's ups and downs. They maintain an ongoing sense of themselves (i.e., as generally the same people they were at thirty) as well as an awareness of improvements and areas of decline. The years have likely provided them with some expertise, some perspective on "how the world works," and some degree of self-acceptance (for better and worse). The years may also have led to a physical or mental slowing down, an increase in irritating aches and pains, and, for some, more trouble concentrating or thinking of the right words to say. However, the age of a person tells us little about his or her individual health, personality, or functioning—any particular 75-year-old could still be working successfully as president of a large corporation or, at the other extreme, could have multiple disabilities requiring nursing home care.

Being 75 also means having been born into a particular historical era and joining a particular generation, or cohort, who shared similar economic, sociocultural, and educational experiences. Marie and the rest of her cohort were raised with an entirely different relationship to the health care system than people born later; they were socialized to view doctors as authority figures who always knew best. With very different notions about mental illness and treatment, they did not often speak openly about emotional concerns and viewed psychiatric care as reserved for those who were truly "crazy."

Further, the generation born in the 1920s lived through events unimaginable to those born later—the Great Depression, World War II, the Cold War—and experienced societal megashifts as well—rapid technological developments, dramatic changes in family structures and communities, and increased ease and frequency of travel. Living through such times undoubtedly influenced their values and attitudes and approaches to solving problems; for example, unquestioning patriotism, frugality, and marital commitment were common ideals for that generation.

Finally, older adults in the United States face certain normative experiences: They are currently likely to become grandparents, exit full-time work roles, have decreased incomes, depend on Medicare or Medicaid for health insurance coverage, and face the loss of spouses, friends, and relatives to disabling illness and death.

What we know now about "aging" and "older people" is based largely on what we have learned from people born early in the twentieth century; of course, what we know about depression in late life is based on research and clinical experience with those same people. Given the complex interplay between adult development and historical context, it is difficult to predict how Baby Boomers and younger generations will experience aging or depressive illness late in life. With the aging population and predictions that rates of mental illness will be higher in subsequent generations of elderly, the need to understand the relationship between aging and depression—and to provide geriatric mental health care—is growing (Jeste et al., 1999).

A Biopsychosocial Theoretical Framework

Depression can be multiply determined, maintained, and treated. Attending to the interplay of biomedical, psychological, social, and systemic factors that affect geriatric depression allows for multiple avenues of intervention—psychotherapy, antidepressant medication, case management programs, and/or some combination of these and other treatments.

Marie's case illustrates the importance of a biopsychosocial conceptualization of factors that relate to her depression. She was recently started on an antihypertensive medication that can cause depressive symptoms, and unstable blood sugars may affect her mood and energy. Also, she has a prior psychiatric history, with one episode of depression in her thirties. For the most part, she has been a woman who coped with stress and loss by taking action and getting involved with work, hobbies, and her community. But her options for such action have decreased with successive losses of her job, her husband, her best friend, and her mobility.

What are the implications of Marie's feeling more dependent and less able to cope through activity? How accessible are her children for help and support? What about her needs for transportation and assistance with chores at home? What is her eligibility for affordable mental health services? What are her needs and wishes for future living arrangements? A comprehensive treatment plan will acknowledge and attempt to address this broad range of issues.

Pragmatic, Relational, and Ethical Considerations

Communication

The critical ingredients for successfully engaging older adults into mental health care are the empathy and skill to communicate with clarity, kindness, and respect. False assumptions about the elderly all too often compromise how clinicians interact with them, however. It pays to question these assumptions.

Imagine visiting a doctor (or other health care professional) you had never met to discuss your concern that you've been uncharacteristically fatigued, and say you decided to bring a friend along for support. Imagine the doctor coming in to the examining room and asking your friend what seems to be the trouble with you. Or, imagine he is talking to you as if you were a child or not very bright.

Or, suppose you had trouble hearing and your doctor seems to be mumbling questions from behind his computer screen. Or, at the other extreme, suppose you could hear quite well but for some reason the doctor is shouting at you. And, how would you feel if you were anxious and thinking kind of slowly and, after being rapidly presented for five minutes with complicated information and treatment options, you were asked to decide which treatment you wanted and felt shy to ask the rushed doctor to explain further?

In general, the golden rule is a fairly good guide for communicating with older patients: Talk to them as you hope a doctor would talk to you. Communication should be adapted according to observations about the individual's capacity to hear and see and grasp information. The reward is discovering, as students new to gerontology do, that even among frail elderly in nursing home settings, each body housing medical and cognitive problems contains an individual with a rich history.

Interprofessional Collaboration

Marie was somewhat unusual for someone of her generation in that she brought her concerns about depressive symptoms directly to the attention of her primary care doctor. The doctor was also somewhat unusual in appreciating the depressive symptoms expressed by his 75-year-old patient and offering her a treatment. However, he could not possibly address all of Marie's contributing problems on his own. Plus, he may not have been aware that she could barely afford the treatment that he did offer. Depending on the most salient concerns, as well as the availability of services, Marie might benefit from consultation with one or more of these professionals: a social worker, psychologist, geriatric psychiatrist, community care nurse, dietician, low-vision rehab specialist, or others.

Good geriatric care often entails interprofessional collaboration, including coordination of care among different providers. In some settings, a geriatric care team is already in place, allowing for an interdisciplinary treatment plan to address the biological, psychological, and social aspects of the elder's care. In many settings, however, such a team does not exist but can be informally put together with a few telephone calls and an attitude of cooperation that says, "How can we help each other to help this patient?" *With the older adult's permission*, referrals can be made and information shared as appropriate.

Advocacy and Outreach

A final theme that guides our work with depressed elders is the relatively active stance we take vis-à-vis our patients' care. This stance most often applies to cases in which the older adult has disabilities that affect her capacity to follow through with recommended treatments. While we never want to "take over" functions that an older adult can do for herself, thus creating unnecessary dependency, we do want to be alert to areas of limited capacity. For example, when an older adult with memory problems does not come in for her medical or mental health appointment, we call to see if she forgot and reschedule. For those who need reminders, we might employ the family's help or, in the absence of such help, call the older adult the morning of her appointment to remind her. This approach is atypical for most care systems, where it is up to the patient to reschedule if they don't show for an appointment.

This active stance is important in considering, for example, the older adult's ability to take medications as directed, to get transportation to appointments, to live safely on her own, to obtain information about alternative medical treatments, and to access various systems of care. If an older client is having problems in any of these areas, we work to determine the cause of the problem and to optimize the client's ability to access care and make decisions consistent with her values.

An important ethical issue in working with frail older adults is to maintain a balance between working to promote the elder's autonomy while at the same time advocating for her safety (Haley and Mangum, 1999). In these situations, a comprehensive evaluation of the older adult's capacity to make rational decisions consistent with her values is necessary (Moye, 1999). In most cases, depressed older adults remain capable of making rational decisions for themselves and we work as their advocates in this context, even if we don't always agree with their decisions. In other cases, depressed elders are not capable of making rational decisions (e.g., due to advanced dementia or psychotic thinking secondary to depression) and in these situations we work as advocates to protect their safety.

The Book

Part I defines late-life depression (Chapter 2) and presents approaches to its assessment and treatment (Chapter 3), all in the context of our commitments to a biopsychosocial framework for conceptualizing it, a respectful relational stance toward the patient, and interprofessional collaboration.

Part II embodies fourteen case studies representing the range of presentations of depression in late life as well as a range of interventions in different care settings. Each is intended to demonstrate the positive potential for improving the older adult's mood, functioning, and quality of life.

The appendices compile practical resources. They review (A) the use of antidepressant medication, (B) recommended assessment tools, (C) new models of integrated geriatric mental health care that promise to improve services, and (D) recommended readings, Web sites, and organizational resources.

CHAPTER TWO

Defining the Problem

Depression in late life takes many forms—in terms of severity, symptoms, and coexisting problems. Especially prevalent among older adults is minor depression, which is frequently experienced in the context of changing physical abilities. Usually, these "minor" depressive symptoms cause further, but avoidable, disability. For example, 82-year-old Bernice doubts she'll walk comfortably again despite successful knee replacement surgery, and she feels it's too much effort to bother with her physical therapy exercises. Brief psychotherapy to address her poor motivation and hopelessness can ultimately help her to walk into town every day as she used to, rather than sit inside feeling useless. At the other extreme, older adults can experience life-threatening psychotic and/or suicidal depression. Joanna stopped eating because she was convinced she no longer had a throat; she required inpatient hospitalization and electroconvulsive therapy to prevent her death (see Chapter 17).

This chapter provides an overview of DSM-IV depressive syndromes and their distinct implications for older adults, as well as of depressive syndromes particular to the geriatric population. It also reviews the risks for and costs of depression in late life. As the case studies in Part II will illustrate, late-life depression and its treatment vary according to coexisting problems (e.g., medical illness, chronic pain, dementia, alcohol abuse, grief, trauma), psychiatric history (e.g., history of depression or bipolar disorder), individual differences (e.g., gender, ethnicity, personality), and treatment setting (e.g., community versus nursing home). Comprehensive assessment, as emphasized in the next chapter, helps to guide a treatment plan that takes into account these various factors.

Prevalence and Cost of the Problem

Defining the extent of "the problem" is not easy and is open to some debate. We do know that the large majority of older adults are *not* depressed. We also know, based on results of the Epidemiological Catchment Area Study of the early 1980s, that a very small minority of older adults (1–2%) suffer from a DSM-III-defined major depressive episode within a given year; this rate is lower than for younger adults (3–4%) (Weissman et al., 1991). A relatively large gray area lies between "no depression" and "major depression." A significant minority of older adults does report high levels of depressive symptoms that do not meet diagnostic criteria. For example, on a self-report depression rating scale, an older adult may admit to having trouble sleeping and concentrating, decreased motivation for activity, and diminished feelings of self-worth, but not have the number, intensity, or severity of symptoms to warrant a major depression diagnosis. From a diagnostic standpoint, these symptoms can reflect a related problem such as dysthymia or an adjustment disorder, or they may not fit neatly into any current diagnostic category. Rates of clinically significant depressive symptoms among older adults range from 10–15% in community settings to 25–30% in inpatient medical and long-term care settings (Blazer, 1994).

Some people argue that subsyndromal depressive symptoms in older adults represent normal, expected discouragement as opposed to a psychiatric condition amenable to treatment. We view this as a complex question. Certainly, late-in-life loss can bring sadness and chronic illness can bring changes in physical or mental activity, and these are normal experiences. On the other hand, depressive symptoms that have a negative impact on the individual's health or functioning (e.g., that lead to the kind of poor self-care that can exacerbate chronic illness), and that have been found by researchers to be amenable to treatment, should be considered "clinically significant."

The evidence is strong that depression, even minor depression, is costly to the individual and the society. In adults of all ages, depression relates to individual suffering, declining physical health, lost work, family burden, and increased health care costs (Johnson, Weissman, and Klerman, 1992; Judd et al., 1996; Wells et al., 1989). Let's look in more detail at the relation of depression to excess functional disability, mortality, increased health service use, and individual suffering among older adults.

Depression causes excess disability in older adults. That is, whatever impact a chronic illness has on an elder's functioning, depression is likely to make it worse (Bruce et al., 1994). Unfortunately, this can create a downward spiral in health, functioning, and quality of life. For example, Bernice–who developed depression in the context of grief and immobility secondary to arthritis and knee surgery–was less motivated to work on her rehabilitation exercises, more sensitive to pain, and more likely to isolate from friends who would normally encourage her. If these changes persist, she will likely become physically weaker and less confident in her ability to feel better, thus the downward spiral. A number of studies have shown that depressed patients are less likely to benefit from rehabilitation in the case of stroke, heart attack, chronic obstructive pulmonary disease, arthritis, hip fracture, and Parkinson's disease (Katz, 1996). Other health implications of depression can include malnutrition, increased sensitivity to pain, and decreased likelihood of following through with prescribed medications or other treatments.

Depression is also associated with increased mortality in late life. Of course, people who are the most sick–and thus at greatest risk of dying–are also at greater risk for depression. However, even when controlling for the severity of physical illness, older adults who are depressed are more likely to die when followed over time; this link may be mediated by physiological (e.g., blood chemistry) and/or behavioral (e.g., poor motivation for self-care) factors (Penninx et al., 1999; Schulz et al., 2000). For example, evidence is growing about the relationship between depression and cardiac illness. Again, controlling for the severity of cardiac illness, patients who are depressed are more likely to die within six months after a heart attack than those who are not depressed (Frasure-Smith, Lesperance, and Talajic, 1993). Recent research actually shows that depressed older adults are at greater risk of developing heart disease in the first place (Ariyo et al., 2000). Finally, older adults who are depressed are at significantly increased risk for mortality through suicide (Conwell et al., 1996, 2000).

Depression is expensive from an economic standpoint. Depressed patients use more health care services, including physician visits, emergency room visits, medications, and inpatient hospital days, than their nondepressed counterparts. That holds among adults of all ages and in cases of both major and minor depression–and not only because they typically have more medical problems. The extra service use is above and beyond the cost of treating the depression (Callahan et al., 1994; Simon, Von Korff, and Barlow, 1995; Unützer et al., 1997).

The greatest human cost of geriatric depression is the suffering of those elders who are depressed. To face the final years of one's life feeling helpless, empty, and hopeless is devastating. To watch one's older mother, father, sibling, or friend suffer from depression–and to live with or care for such an elder–is similarly difficult. The individual, interpersonal, and economic reasons for preventing and treating depression in late life are multiple.

Challenges for Recognizing Late-Life Depression

Despite the prevalence and cost of the problem, depression is frequently not recognized and, thus, not treated in older people. There are many reasons for this oversight, including the biases of clinicians and of elders themselves, misattribution of symptoms, and the actual complexity of diagnosing depression in some medically or neurologically ill elders.

Older adults, families, and health care professionals often assume that it is reasonable or expectable for old people to be depressed (e.g., less active, less engaged, more somatically preoccupied). Therefore, their symptoms may not be seen as problems amenable to help. Moreover, the losses that some elders face can inspire feelings of helplessness and hopelessness in their care providers; it can seem a lot easier not to "go there."

Sorting out medical from psychological symptoms is difficult in some elders. Often, depressed elders do not conceptualize their distress in psychological or psychiatric terms. A depressed 86-year-old Samuel may tell his doctor "I feel lousy," rather than "I feel depressed" (or anxious, or worthless, or agitated). Or, when asked how he is feeling, he might stick with his proud, "not great, doc, but you take one day at a time."

Further, somatic depressive symptoms—such as fatigue, insomnia, changes in concentration or memory—are commonly attributed by clinicians to medical or neurological illness in an older person. These difficulties are exaggerated for older adults who have lengthy medical histories, multiple symptoms, complex medication regimens, and/or cognitive changes. As we discuss in the next chapter, we need to ask older adults with vague or multiple somatic complaints very specific questions about their mood, outlook, and behavior. For those with limited insight or verbal capacity, we need to ask these questions of their family or caregivers.

Extensive research has been and is being conducted on how to improve clinicians' recognition of geriatric depression, especially in primary care settings. Because most older adults do not self-refer to mental health professionals, medical care settings represent the best opportunity to recognize and connect depressed elders to appropriate treatment. We discuss issues of depression screening and models of care integration further in Chapter 3 and Appendices C and D.

DSM-IV Depressive Syndromes in the Elderly

At the time of this writing, the DSM-IV (American Psychiatric Association, 1994) is generally used to guide psychiatric diagnosis for purposes of treatment planning and billing/reimbursement. Symptoms of depression in older adults are often consistent with diagnostic criteria for one of the DSM-IV affective disorders, including major depressive disorder, bipolar disorder, dysthymic disorder, depression secondary to other conditions (medical illness or substance use), or an adjustment disorder or bereavement. In other cases, depressive symptoms in an older adult do not neatly fit one of these diagnostic entities, and such individuals may ultimately receive a working diagnosis of "Depressive Disorder Not Otherwise Specified (NOS)." Frequently, depressive symptoms are related to other medical or psychiatric disorders, such as dementia, substance abuse, anxiety disorders, or personality disorders. These differential diagnostic issues will be addressed in the case study discussions in Part II.

Here, we first review special considerations for using DSM-IV affective disorder diagnostic categories with older adults and then discuss the subsyndromal depressive conditions that appear to have special relevance to this population.

Major Depressive Disorder

Diagnosing major depression in an older adult is often straightforward. A relatively healthy older adult can have clear symptoms and functional changes of major depression, without complex differential diagnostic questions. In older adults with medical/neurological problems, or with otherwise atypical presentations, establishing a major depression diagnosis can be trickier.

Somatic Symptoms. How do you know if somatic symptoms–appetite and/or weight changes, insomnia or hypersomnia, fatigue or loss of energy, psychomotor retardation or agitation, diminished concentration–suggest major depression, or are symptomatic of a patient's medical illness or illnesses? For example, an 83-year-old man with coronary artery disease and congestive heart failure is tiring very easily at his part-time grocery bagging job, is having trouble concentrating on his weekly newsmagazine, has trouble sitting still at home, is yelling at his wife more than usual, and is waking several times during the night. Should these symptoms–assuming he also admits to changes in his mood or interest–count toward a depression diagnosis?

According to DSM-IV, somatic symptoms count toward a major depressive disorder diagnosis unless they are "clearly and fully accounted for by a general medical condition" (p. 323). For example, weight loss occurring during a month of chronic diarrhea would be attributed to the medical condition, whereas increased fatigue in the context of a chronic medical condition would be counted toward a depression diagnosis if its cause were not absolutely clear. A comprehensive evaluation of the timing, nature, and clustering of symptoms, as well as signs of functional changes in usual activity or relationships, helps to sort this out. The clinician must be aware of two possible biases: attributing all somatic complaints to medical causes in older adults, thus underdiagnosing depression, and attributing all somatic complaints to psychiatric causes in older adults, thus overdiagnosing depression and possibly overlooking changes in physical health status.

Cognitive Symptoms. DSM-IV notes that: "In elderly adults, cognitive symptoms (e.g., disorientation, memory loss, and distractibility) may be particularly prominent" features of major depression (p. 325). Memory complaints in an older person may be mistaken for signs of dementia when they are really symptomatic of depression. Active complaints about memory problems are more common in depression than in dementia, given the limited insight into memory loss frequently seen in dementia. Again, a comprehensive evaluation–often including neuropsychological testing–helps to sort out the diagnostic significance of concentration or memory changes in an older adult.

Affective Symptoms. The current cohort of older adults tends to minimize emotional distress based on the sociocultural norms of their upbringing. In particular, older men are less likely than older women to express vulnerable emotions; the same is true of ethnic versus nonethnic elders. In addition, in older adults, clinical depression can occur without the experience of sadness (Gallo et al., 1997); loss of interest or pleasure and/or loss of motivation may be more common in these cases (Forsell, Jorm, and Winblad, 1994). Therefore, in screening for depression (see Chapter 3), it is important to frame mood questions with variants of, "Are you feeling sad or depressed?" such as: "How are your spirits these days?" "What have you enjoyed doing lately?" "Do you often get bored?" "Do you feel helpless?" "Do you feel that your life is empty?" "Do you worry too much?" (Hoyl et al., 1999; Reynolds and Kupfer, 1999).

Functional Changes. The diagnosis of major depressive disorder requires that symptoms cause significant distress or impairment in social, occupational, or other areas of functioning. Impaired functioning may be harder to detect in an older adult with multiple chronic illnesses and who no longer works and spends most of her time at home. To uncover significant functional decline, it is therefore helpful to ask older adults specifically about changes in their typical activities–about hygiene and grooming, telephone calls, reading or television viewing, keeping up with chores at home, hobbies, family or social visiting, church attendance, taking medications, or performing other regular health behaviors such as checking blood sugars. Has the individual, or a close observer, noticed any difference in her ability to function in these areas?

Beyond DSM. Major depression manifests itself in some older adults with symptoms that are not among DSM-IV criteria. As mentioned above, apathy or amotivation is a common symptom of depression in older adults; complicating matters is the fact that apathy is also common in dementia. Irritability is frequently a sign of depression in older men. Excessive physical complaints are common, and can reflect the exacerbation of physical maladies or pain by depression, and/or the somatic expression of emotional distress. [Men commonly cite stomach complaints, burning with urination, palpitations, and shortness of breath (Koenig et al., 1993).] Anxious rumination and other anxiety symptoms are also characteristic of late-life depression (Blazer, Hughes, and Fowler, 1989; Parmalee, Katz, and Lawton, 1993).

Other Features. Major depressive disorder varies in severity, recurrence, and the presence or absence of psychotic features in adults of all ages. Older adults can experience it in late life for the first time, or as a recurrence of an earlier illness. Since understanding prior patterns and risks for depression can aid current treatment, it is important to obtain a thorough psychiatric history. Older adults may be at higher risk for major depression with psychotic features (Blazer and Koenig, 1996), frequently with delusions of persecution or an incurable illness–most often related to the abdomen (e.g., gastrointestinal cancer), as in the case of a 78-year-old man who stopped eating because he believed food could not travel through him. Finally, suicidal thoughts are common in depressed elders. It is critical to differentiate normative thoughts about death and dying from thoughts or plans to take one's own life.

Bipolar and Manic Depression

Major depression in an older adult sometimes occurs as an episode of a bipolar disorder, so it is a good idea to inquire about histories of mania, hypomania, or treatment for bipolar disorder.

Mania appears to be relatively uncommon among older adults (Weissman et al., 1991), although a fair number of chronically mentally ill elders are long survivors of bipolar illness and can continue to experience manic episodes (Meeks, 1999; Young and Klerman, 1992). The case of Elaine (Chapter 16) reveals a strong family history of bipolar disorder and a personal history of depression and hypomanic episodes preceding a first manic episode in late life.

First onset of mania in late life, in the absence of a history of affective disorder, is likely to have organic roots (Young and Klerman, 1992). Manic symptoms can present secondary to medical and neurological problems (particularly cerebrovascular and other brain diseases), medications, or drugs of abuse. A case in point is the 79-year-old woman with no history of psychiatric illness who takes high doses of prednisone to treat her pulmonary disease: One morning, her neighbor found her sitting naked and digging through her garden, eagerly "looking for ancient remains"–she was diagnosed with steroid toxicity and hospitalized.

Antidepressant medications can also cause manic episodes in some older adults. For instance, a 75-year-old man with a hypomanic personality style at baseline and a family history of bipolar disorder developed mania when given fluoxetine (Prozac) to treat his depression. He required a brief inpatient hospital stay to change his medication regimen to help stabilize his mood.

According to DSM-IV, older adults with bipolar illness commonly experience mixed episodes, with symptoms of both mania and major depression. Older manic patients may present, therefore, with dysphoria, and symptoms including agitation, insomnia, appetite dysregulation, psychotic features, and suicidal thinking. Some studies suggest that older adults are at greater risk for more frequent relapse/cycling of bipolar affective episodes.

Dysthymic Disorder

A diagnosis of dysthymia requires the persistence of depressed mood and two of six additional depressive symptoms for more than two years. Some dysthymic older adults report a lifetime of mild depression and self-doubt, while others report symptoms starting only in later years. From a psychological standpoint, late-onset dysthymia may reflect a loss of self-esteem resulting from a sense of diminished control over one's abilities and usual coping strategies (Blazer and Koenig, 1996). From a cultural perspective, older adults in a society that emphasizes action and productivity may develop chronic depressive symptoms when losing a sense of recognition or purpose. However, dysthymia is not a usual consequence of aging; most older adults who develop disabling chronic illness do not develop dysthymia or other affective disorders.

Dysthymia appears to manifest differently in older and younger people (Devanand et al., 1994; Kirby et al., 1999). Older adults with dysthymia are less likely to have other psychiatric or personality disorders and more likely to have a late age of onset (i.e., fifties or sixties) related to major life stressors and medical illness/disability. Symptoms are cognitive and affective rather than vegetative, and patients present with prominent anxiety, loss of interest, and negative views of themselves and the future. The case of Theresa in Chapter 6 illustrates dysthymia as experienced by a woman with long-standing self-doubt, exacerbated by increased isolation, boredom, and pain.

Depression Secondary to Other Conditions

An older woman suffers a stroke and develops chronic depression. A man is started on an antihypertensive medication and becomes disinterested and depressed. A woman taking steroids for her rheumatoid arthritis develops mania. In these cases, a mood disorder results directly from a medical condition or the effect of substance use or withdrawal. The mood changes are not reactive to the stress of having an illness, but rather are a direct physiological consequence of the condition through neurochemical or structural pathways. Illnesses such as stroke, heart attack, Alzheimer's disease, Parkinson's disease, multiple sclerosis, pancreatic cancer, hypothyroidism, Cushing's disease, and vitamin B-12 deficiency can cause depression, as can medications such as certain antihypertensives (e.g., methyldopa, reserpine, beta blockers), ulcer drugs (e.g., cimetidine), steroids (e.g., prednisone), seizure drugs (e.g., phenobarbital), cancer chemotherapy drugs, benzodiazepines and other sedative drugs or alcohol, and opioid (narcotic) pain medications.

The assessment of depression in older adults should take into account the time of use or discontinuation of medications and timing of onset of medical disorders. The process benefits from collaboration with the patients' medical care providers, as the next chapter elucidates.

Adjustment Disorder

An adjustment disorder is a "maladaptive reaction to an identifiable stressor" (DSM-IV), and can present with symptoms of depression, anxiety, and/or other behavioral disturbance. Given the chronic nature of many of the stressors in the lives of older adults (e.g., physical disability, social isolation, caregiving), it can be difficult to sort out an adjustment disorder from dysthymia and minor depression (see below). It is a useful conceptualization when an older adult develops symptoms of depression/anxiety in response to a new stress, but does not suffer the number or severity of cognitive and vegetative (e.g., changes in energy, sleep, appetite) symptoms that would meet criteria for a major depressive disorder. Adjustment disorders may be specified as acute or chronic, and they may be diagnosed as chronic if they occur in response to chronic stressors (American Psychiatric Association, 1994).

Bereavement

Older adults frequently lose loved ones, and many suffer normal bereavement reactions–which can include depressed mood, crying, sleep disturbance, appetite loss, and trouble concentrating. Bereavement is considered neither a depressive disorder nor an adjustment disorder; in fact, it is not considered a disorder at all unless severe symptoms persist beyond several months and become functionally disabling, at which point a depressive disorder may be diagnosed. The relationship among bereavement, complicated grief, and depression is illustrated in the case of Pauline Feld (Chapter 5), who had persisting depressive symptoms for two years following her husband's death.

Other Depressive Syndromes in the Elderly

Depressive symptoms in older adults are frequently difficult to categorize from a diagnostic perspective. In some cases, symptoms are not severe or enduring enough to meet criteria for the disorders described above. As such, "minor depression" is receiving a lot of attention as an important clinical entity among older adults—but it is difficult to distinguish from chronic adjustment disorder or, if enduring enough, dysthymia, when older adults experience depressive symptoms in response to changes in their abilities or relationships. Further, older adults may experience significant overlap between symptoms of depression and anxiety and between depressive and neurological symptoms. Many people with late-onset depression may have concurrent cerebrovascular disease and a syndrome of "vascular depression" has been proposed in older adults (see below).

Minor Depression

Minor depression, not yet classified by DSM-IV as a distinct disorder but listed as a proposed disorder, entails "one or more periods of depressive symptoms that are identical to Major Depressive Episodes in duration, but which involve fewer symptoms and less impairment" (p. 719). The diagnosis would require at least two of the symptoms of major depression (one of which must be depressed mood or diminished interest) for at least a two-week period.

One study of minor, or subthreshold, depression in the elderly found that many people with depressive symptoms "missed" the diagnostic criteria for major depression by one or two symptoms and those for dysthymia because symptoms had not endured long enough (nearly every day for at least two years) (Gieselmann and Bauer, 2000). In addition to these quantitative differences, symptomatic patterns differed between those with subthreshold depressive symptoms and those with major depression; the former were significantly less likely to report insomnia, feelings of guilt or worthlessness, or suicidal thoughts, but did report similar levels of subjective distress in response to questions about life satisfaction and perceived health.

The case of Eleanor, a healthy, 92-year-old woman with failing vision (Chapter 4), illustrates the importance of recognizing and treating minor, subsyndromal depressive symptoms in an older adult. She became disabled by decreased motivation and social withdrawal and was helped by a group therapy intervention.

Vascular Depression

"Vascular depression" is hypothesized to represent a subtype of late-onset depression (Alexopoulos et al., 1997). Older adults with vascular diseases, including hypertension, coronary artery disease, stroke, and vascular dementia, have relatively high rates of depression. Conversely, adults with late-onset depression have relatively high rates of cerebrovascular disease and related cognitive impairments.

Vascular disease in the brain, caused by arteriosclerotic changes in cerebral blood vessels, can consist of tiny lesions (often in subcortical and frontal regions) occurring without obvious behavioral signs or can result in stroke with obvious motor, speech, or cognitive changes. Cerebrovascular disease and depression appear to co-occur. In cases of vascular dementia–where the individual suffers from functionally significant changes in memory and other cognitive abilities–depression is quite common. Cognitive deficits in executive functioning in particular (planning, initiating, and organizing activity, and abstracting) are common, and depressed older adults with executive dysfunction are more likely to experience relapse and recurrence of depression (Alexopoulos et al., 2000).

Our clinical experience in the VA medical centers, where many older veterans suffer from vascular diseases, is consistent with this emerging research literature. In the face of multiple medical risk factors, these veterans often experience late-onset depression characterized by amotivation, psychomotor retardation, and poor initiative, but less intense depressive ideation such as guilt or worthlessness–except expression of discouragement about their difficulty motivating themselves for activity. This clinical picture fits with Alexopoulos's description of vascular depression (Alexopoulos et al., 1997) and is illustrated by George's case in Chapter 11.

Mixed Anxiety-Depressive Disorder

Symptoms of depression and anxiety commonly overlap, such that disorders can be difficult to distinguish. For example, a ruminative, worried, somatically preoccupied, helpless, hopeless presentation in an older adult has key features of both depression and generalized anxiety, as the cases of Arnie (Chapter 8) and Geneva (Chapter 10) illustrate. In proposing this diagnostic category for consideration, DSM-IV reviews it as a syndrome common in primary care and outpatient mental health settings (but not particular to older adults); the syndrome entails distressing or disabling symptoms of both anxiety and depression, but does not meet criteria for any other disorder.

Common Comorbidities

Depressed older adults often have one or more other medical, neurological, or psychiatric problems. As we have emphasized, geriatric depression often occurs in the context of medical illness, and depression commonly co-occurs with dementia and/or anxiety. In addition, it is important to consider the potential role of substance abuse (e.g., alcohol, benzodiazepines), personality disorder, posttraumatic stress disorder, or grief as related to depression in an older patient. Finally, late-life depression can relate to a wide range of psychosocial stresses that may be amenable to intervention. The case studies in Part II illustrate many of the depressive syndromes described above, as well as common medical, psychiatric, and psychosocial comorbidities.

Diversity: Gender, Ethnicity, and Other Variables

Generalizing about "depression in late life" runs the risk of overlooking the very wide diversity among older adults. First, "older adults" comprise several generations, that is, people ranging in age from the early sixties to over one hundred years. And, our understanding of interactions among age, gender, and ethnicity, for example, remains limited (Haley, Han, and Henderson, 1998; Koenig et al., 1992; Morales, 1999; Steffens et al., 1997; Weissman et al., 1991). Here are some important issues to consider:

- *Differential risks.* For example, women are at higher risk for depression across the life span, men are far more likely to commit suicide in late life, and older Hispanics have higher rates of depression than older Caucasians or African-Americans.

- *Different presentations.* For example, certain socioethnic groups (e.g., less acculturated Hispanic and Asian elders in the United States) may describe depressive symptoms more somatically.
- *Different levels of comfort with exposing vulnerability.* For example, African-American men are comparatively unlikely to admit to negative thoughts or feelings, although it is not clear whether they actually experience less depression or just report less.
- *Reliability of screening tools across groups.* The norms for many measurement scales derive from mostly white samples. Also, when translations of scales are not validated, accurate screening of those whose primary language is not English may well be compromised.
- *Differential use of medical and mental health care services.* For example, less acculturated ethnic elders are more likely to turn to their families for support and are less inclined to seek formal care services. Many have faced a history of discrimination by the health care system and may maintain understandable distrust.
- *Individuality.* Apart from such broad demographic distinctions, each older person has her own personal and family history, intellectual capacity, personality style, relationship experiences, and spiritual involvements, all of which influence ways of coping with stress and expressing distress.
- *Age alone tells us little.*

Risk Factors: Who Gets Depressed in Late Life?

Risk for depression, at any age, is commonly understood to entail an interaction among biomedical, psychological, and social influences. Like many illnesses, depression can be viewed to occur in the context of both an individual's vulnerability or predisposition to it—biological (genetic, medical, neurological) or psychological (personality, coping style)—and environmental factors triggering onset, among them socioeconomic factors, interpersonal loss or conflict, or other life circumstances that challenge the ability to cope or sustain a sense of control.

Of course, these vulnerabilities and stresses interact in complex ways. For example, individuals with certain personality styles are more likely to experience interpersonal conflict. Or, certain economic conditions put individuals at greater risk for medical vulnerability to depression. In addition, depression itself influences these vulnerabilities and stresses: It often leads to or exacerbates interpersonal problems and complicates medical illness.

The relative influence of the various biological, psychological, and social factors on the onset of depression may change across the life span (Karel, 1997). We know that older adults are at greater risk owing to biomedical factors (e.g., vascular disease), whereas psychological vulnerability may be more salient among younger adults. Risk factors also differ for early- and late-onset depression (Alexopoulos et al., 1988b), for major and minor depression (Beekman et al., 1995), and for other depressive syndromes (e.g., Newmann et al., 1996). By reviewing key biological, psychological, and social risk factors for depression in older adults (Fiske, Kasl-Godley, and Gatz, 1998; George, 1994; Karel, 1997), we can identify high-risk groups and target our clinical outreach and screening efforts accordingly. From the perspective of the individual case, isolating risk factors guides assessment and treatment planning.

Biological Risk

Genetic factors play at least some role in the etiology of affective disorders, especially bipolar illness. Evidence suggests that they weigh more heavily in early-onset than in late-onset depression. From the standpoint of risk assessment, it is important to know about an older adult's family history of psychiatric illness, including depression, psychotic disorders, substance abuse, and suicidality. It is also helpful to know what treatments were helpful to family members with similar problems.

While the stress of having an illness or disability constitutes a significant risk for late-life depression (see below), there are also biological links between certain illnesses of late life—especially neurological, vascular, and endocrine diseases—and the onset of depression (see the earlier section "Depression Secondary to Other Conditions"). Also, persisting insomnia, not uncommon in older adults, can lead to depression, as can chronic pain; some older adults experience a vicious cycle of pain, insomnia, and depression (Chapter 9). Because many medications can cause or exacerbate depression, their potential impact must always be ruled out. The same is true of alcohol and other illicit drug use.

Psychological Risk

Personality factors, cognitive schemas regarding sense of control and self-efficacy, and coping styles all relate to an individual's risk for developing depression. As we grow older, we tend to bring our personalities and coping styles along with us. Many of us become, if anything, psychologically stronger: Development through adulthood appears to offer older adults greater self-acceptance, and greater capacities to cope adaptively with stress (with less emotional reactivity, greater thoughtfulness, less self-blame) and to maintain a sense of control even in the face of losses. On an individual basis, however, older adults who have always been prone to dysphoria and self-doubt, who suffer from certain personality disorders, or who are unable to show flexibility in coping strategies as their abilities change are at greater risk of suffering from depression. Trauma, for example, in early or later life, often continues to influence one's worldview and coping style.

The ability to adapt one's coping strategies appears to be particularly important for positive mental health in later years. For a simple example, if a man can no longer shovel the driveway after a snowstorm, he is less likely to feel helpless and distressed if he can adjust his expectations of himself (it's OK to be able to shovel the front stoop but not the entire driveway), can ask for help from a grandson or neighbor, or can feel grateful that he is able to walk slowly even if he lacks the strength to shovel the driveway (Heckhausen and Schulz, 1993). In contrast, imagine a 78-year-old man who struggled since childhood with dysthymia, but generally maintained his spirits through lifting weights—until cardiac surgery at the age of 72 reduced his stamina for lifting as much or as long, and he became quite depressed. Not being able to shovel the driveway aroused a profound sense of helplessness and worthlessness in this man, who could not alter his expectations or consider alternative strategies for maintaining his sense of self-esteem, and so was psychologically at risk for late-life depression.

Stress and Social Factors

At all ages, women are at higher risk for depression. This gender gap remains throughout life, although there is some evidence that it may narrow in very old age. Race does not appear to be a strong predictor, but limited educational background and chronic financial strain do. As does marriage: Married older adults are at lower risk for depression than those who are not; divorced or separated elderly are at greatest risk.

The stress most predictive of depression in late life is physical disability. While biochemical and neurological factors linking illness to depression are important, it is the impact of illness on one's abilities–and on one's sense of self, control, and purpose–that correlates most strongly.

Interpersonal stress and loss are also sources of risk; conversely, relationships and positive transitions can be protective against depression. While most older adults who suffer the death of a loved one do not become clinically depressed, bereavement does pose increased risk for some. Being a caregiver to a physically, cognitively, and/or emotionally impaired elder is an important risk, as are social isolation and conflictual relationships. Protective social factors include social support–including contact with others and instrumental and emotional help as needed–and religious or spiritual involvement.

Life events or transitions–such as retirement or relocation–can pose risk for depression or contribute to happiness and adaptive coping, depending on the individual's sense of control over and personal meaning of the event.

Summary

Depression in late life comes in many forms and with many causes. What is common to depressive syndromes in late life is their contribution to individual and family suffering, excess disability, and societal cost. Treatable depression is frequently not identified as such by elders, their families, or their health care providers. Overcoming age-related biases, improving professional and public awareness about geriatric mental health concerns, and designing good models of care (see Appendix C) are necessary for connecting depressed older adults to effective treatments. The next chapter reviews strategies for assessing late-life depression and the range of treatment approaches that can help.

CHAPTER THREE

Perspectives on Assessment and Treatment

During his annual physical exam, 78-year-old Bill Jones was reserved and polite with his primary care doctor. He had suffered a stroke two years ago, about a year after the death of his wife of 52 years. Having to give up driving and needing extra help at the time, he sold and moved out of his house to live with his daughter Jean and her family. Bill's physical exam and labs confirmed that, apart from his residual right-sided weakness, slow speech, and moderate hearing loss, his health was stable. When asked how he was doing, Bill told the doctor, "I'm bored and sometimes I think I'm losing my marbles, but I manage. My kids are always worrying about me, but I'm almost 80, so what should I expect?" The doctor asked, "Are you feeling depressed?" Bill replied that he was fine and wished his kids wouldn't worry so much. They scheduled his follow-up appointment for six months later.

Before a comprehensive mental health evaluation can occur, someone has to identify a possible problem. As in Bill's case, that "someone" is often the primary care provider (PCP). Even if the older person or his family suspects a problem with depression, it is often the PCP whom they initially consult. The PCP has a difficult job: She has to consider, in 10–20 minutes, the various underlying conditions that could be causing the multiple signs and symptoms presented by her older patients and to initiate treatment as indicated. If depression is suspected, a brief depression screening should be conducted. Such screening can be administered in a range of medical, social, or residential care settings.

A positive screening suggests that the patient may benefit from a more comprehensive psychogeriatric evaluation, which helps to determine whether depression and/or other medical or psychiatric problems exist, and to conceptualize the biomedical, psychological, and social issues that are causing or maintaining them. The conceptualization also guides the initial treatment plan.

In this chapter, we first review general issues for assessing geriatric depression, including the importance of screening, building rapport, and conducting a clinical interview. We then review a repertoire of traditional interventions (e.g., antidepressant medication and evidence-based psychotherapies) as well as general approaches critical to successful intervention with depressed elderly (e.g., role flexibility, care coordination). We emphasize that treatment is a *process* that needs to be monitored and adjusted in approach or intensity over time.

Assessment: Screening for Depression

The first stage in conducting an assessment for depression is recognizing the possibility of a problem. Though such recognition may come from the older adult herself, who notices a change in her own mood, attitude, or functioning, self-referral to mental health treatment is the exception and occurs chiefly among relatively educated, affluent elderly and/or those with prior exposure to mental health services.

More common is the older adult who presents in a medical setting with complaints of not feeling well—but without actually identifying herself as "depressed"—or the older adult who says nothing at all about not feeling well. Frequently, family members bring concerns about the depressed older adult to the attention of medical care providers. They may or may not define their concerns as matters of mental health; comments range from "I think mom is depressed" to "Mom is sleeping more than usual" or "Mom is driving us crazy with her complaints."

Obstacles to Depression Screening

While any such comments should flag a patient for a depression screen, a number of obstacles consistently get in the way. (Note that Bill's doctor did inquire about possible depression, but did not follow up with additional questions—Why were Bill's kids worried about him? Why did Bill think he was "losing his marbles"?). Common barriers to adequate screening include emotional discomfort on the parts of patient and practitioner alike, trouble getting around social norms for communicating with elders, time constraints, and access to further evaluation and treatment (Unützer et al., 1999).

Our Own Discomfort. We are often uncomfortable asking an older patient about feelings of sadness, hopelessness, or suicidality. The discomfort can come from our own sense of helplessness about "What to do" with an older person who seems helpless or distressed. Further, if we don't think there is anything to do to alleviate the distress, we're less likely to inquire about it. When we feel stuck with a problem we are not prepared to address—perhaps because no mental health services exist on site or no easy referral mechanisms are in place—it may seem a lot easier simply to avoid asking an older adult questions that could elicit symptoms of depression.

Communication and Cohort. Older adults and health care providers are likely to have indirect, or incomplete, communication, which complicates matters. People born before about 1930 and those with less education or mainstream acculturation were socialized into a paternalistic medical system and often take a passive stance during a medical encounter. They tend to answer only those questions that are asked and to accept physician authority with little questioning or interaction. Norms for respectful interaction with our elders may render care providers more polite and less direct, and thus less willing to ask about emotional difficulties, substance use, sexual concerns, or other sensitive topics.

One recent study revealed that young physicians were less apt to provide counseling and health education and more disposed to engage in "chatting" and compliance-checking with their older patients (Callahan et al., 2000). Such a friendly visit may also be superficial. "If the unstated rules of social interaction protect older patients from the intrusiveness of others, older patients may be less apt to have all of their health needs identified and addressed, a conclusion with serious implications for quality of care" (p. 33). The result is missed opportunities for recognizing and treating depression in this population.

Time Constraints. Medical settings are very rushed these days. The primary care physician or nurse is responsible for addressing acute and chronic problems as well as a wide range of preventive health issues. Providers may feel that time does not allow for depression evaluation. For complex geriatric patients, this time crunch may be even more difficult (Glasser and Gravdal, 1997). As one patient recently complained, "It takes 30 minutes for my doctor just to write out all my prescriptions!"

Systemic Barriers to Screening Follow-up. A screening is only as good as the procedures in place for following up. When geriatric depression is recognized in primary care settings, it may never be further evaluated or treatment, if initiated (usually a prescription for antidepressant medication), may not be adequately followed up (Bartels et al., 1997; Unützer et al., 2000). In the context of an initial screening, asking further questions as needed is critical, especially regarding risk assessment. For example, if a patient like Bill were to admit to feeling his life is empty and hopeless, the next step would be to ask him if he had any thoughts of suicide. (See Chapter 7 for an example of asking such follow-up questions.)

In general, procedures need to be in place to facilitate referral of a patient for further evaluation and treatment. The extended evaluation may occur by the screener (e.g., the primary care provider) if time and expertise allow, by a mental health specialist on site, or by referral to a specialist. Mechanisms to follow-up on the referral are critical: Simply giving a depressed older adult a slip of paper with the name and phone number of a geriatric psychiatrist often does not result in a contact (for many reasons, not the least of which has been limited Medicare coverage for mental health services). In any event, depressive symptoms in an individual identified as at risk should be monitored over time. Appendix C presents various models of care integration being studied to improve the provision of geriatric mental health services in primary care.

Using Screening Tools

Some of the obstacles to adequate depression screening can be addressed by using structured screening tools. They help because:

- Many care providers do not know or recall the key features of depression that should be assessed.
- They provide an efficient, time-effective way to inquire about depressive symptoms.
- Having a screening questionnaire or interview puts both provider and patient more at ease by way of normalizing the assessment ("We check all of our patients for symptoms of depression/stress, so now it's time to see what concerns you may have along those lines").
- Screenings can be tailored to address a range of preventive health issues, including smoking, alcohol use, seat belt use, completion of advance directives (e.g., health care proxies or living wills), and so forth.
- Research has demonstrated the reliability and validity of several scales for detecting probable depression in older adults.

Screening instruments are not intended to be used alone as diagnostic tools; they are designed so that a certain "cutoff" score is associated with the *probable* presence of clinically significant depression. Appendix B discusses depression scales that are appropriate for screening older adults.

Assessment: Clinical Interview

Once an older adult has been identified as possibly depressed–by herself, her family, her medical doctor, through a formal screening process, or otherwise (e.g., in the context of exploring alcohol use or a cognitive or functional change)–a comprehensive evaluation allows confirmation of a diagnosis and development of an initial treatment plan. The psychogeriatric evaluation, like any other mental health assessment, has several goals:

- To clarify the patient's presenting symptoms and determine a differential diagnosis.
- To identify biological, psychological, and social risk factors that may be causing or maintaining depression in the individual.

- To understand functional implications and possible risks associated with the individual's condition. (Can the person adequately care for him or herself at home?)
- To assess internal and external resources available to help in treatment planning–for example, hobbies that can be rejuvenated, a religious faith that has been a source of strength, the intellectual/emotional capacity to explore the meaning of recent losses, a network of family or friends to help with practical or emotional support, the financial means to cover treatment costs.
- To develop an initial treatment plan in keeping with the conceptualization of the problem.

The way we conduct the process of such an evaluation is no less important than the substantive knowledge we bring regarding geriatric syndromes, risks for depression, and appropriate questions to ask. The capacity to communicate clearly, empathically, and respectfully with the older adult will increase the effectiveness of the initial interview. Beyond the initial interview, assessment is an ongoing activity if treatment is initiated. Throughout the course of treatment, we continue to gather information that may modify our conceptualization of the problem. We continue also to monitor the patient's response to treatment, attending to both signs of improvement and signs of increased depression or other medical/psychiatric difficulties.

Communication Issues

Many older adults feel anxiety or reluctance about participating in an evaluation with a mental health professional. Creating an environment of genuine respect and reassurance will help put them at ease and help the interviewer obtain information necessary to arrive at an accurate working diagnostic impression. Although in many settings time pressure is a reality, the fact remains that a thorough evaluation of an older adult with possible depression or other neuropsychiatric problems cannot be completed in 10–15 minutes; allotting an hour (sometimes more when there are multiple informants) is standard practice.

Interviewing is an art. Depending on an elder's cognitive and interpersonal style, it may be more or less difficult to keep the interview "on track" to obtain the necessary history. Doing just that without appearing rushed, impatient, or disrespectful requires practice as well as commitment to a relational style of interviewing whereby, in our experience, the "best" information emerges. By following Bill's case, we can see the importance of the interview style and setting (as well as family persistence).

> Bill returned to his primary care doctor four months later in the company of his daughter Jean, who had herself called to schedule the appointment because she was worried about her father. She reported that, for the past 5–6 months, he had become increasingly withdrawn and irritable; he was not following recommendations about his diet and use of alcohol, and expressed to the family that things would be better if he weren't a burden to them. When questioned by the doctor, Bill replied that he was fine and that his daughter always worried too much. He said he had no interest in going out to a senior center or other day program, and was content to stay home alone and watch TV. The physician was concerned by Jean's description of his behavior, and made a referral to the local geropsychologist for further evaluation.
>
> Bill and his daughter arrived on time for that appointment a week later, although Jean said that he had tried to convince her that it had been cancelled. The psychologist introduced herself to both of them and asked if Mr. Jones would prefer to come in alone or to have his daughter join him. He said he preferred to have his daughter join him.
>
> The psychologist attempted to normalize the use of her services by older patients who are dealing with stressful changes in their lives. She asked him how he had been doing, and he initially answered, "I'm fine, it's her who is worried." He spoke slowly and with some difficulty, but was easily understood. The psychologist asked Mr. Jones if she could ask his daughter about her concerns and, when he agreed, Jean detailed her worries.

> The psychologist then commented that he and his daughter appeared to have a difference in opinion. In everyday, empathic, simple language, the psychologist remarked to Bill that she would imagine going through all the changes he'd been through would take quite a toll on just about anyone. He agreed. When asked what had been most difficult for him, he became tearful and said he was afraid he was losing his memory.
>
> He was willing to participate in the rest of the evaluation, thanks to the respect shown for his opinion, allowance of sufficient time for him to respond to questions, recognition and normalization of the stress he had experienced, and the use of simple humor and compassion to engage him.

This approach illustrates the importance of respect and making an effort to form an alliance with the older adult. A rushed, authoritative interviewer who prematurely allied with the daughter may not have elicited the trust that enabled this gentleman to disclose how vulnerable he had been feeling. Here, we list several guidelines for conducting a respectful and effective psychogeriatric interview.

- *Obtain permission from the identified elder patient* to include an accompanying family member in the interview, or to invite family's input after the first one-on-one meeting. Do not presume that it is automatically alright to do either.
- *Maximize the older individual's ability to see and hear you.* Hints: Draw up a chair so that you can sit close rather than at a distance or behind a large desk; ask the patient if she can hear you; ask whether one ear is better than the other and, if she has a hearing aid, ask if it is on; try to meet in a setting that minimizes outside noise and distraction; speak loudly if necessary–but be careful not to speak *too* loudly if the person has no hearing deficit. (Note: New trainees, wanting to sound empathic to their clients, frequently talk so softly that their words are not intelligible; with practice, we learn to communicate a sense of caring while speaking clearly and audibly.)

- *Phrase questions simply,* avoiding long complex sentences, if there is evidence of hearing impairment or cognitive deficit. Similarly, avoid speaking too quickly.
- *When a family member joins an interview, address the elder.* Do not refer to him as if he is not there, even if cognitive impairment is suspected. *An older adult with mild to moderate dementia rarely loses the capacity to feel included or excluded from a conversation.* If he has difficulty providing meaningful answers to questions, then ask his permission to obtain information from the other person. Make an effort to continue eye contact with the elder and include him by interjecting humor or acknowledging his accomplishments, grandchildren, and so on.
- *Educate the older adult (and family, if present) about your professional role and the purpose of the interview.* Try to normalize the process and preempt such common fears/fantasies as the assumption that the point of the meeting is to arrange for institutional care in a nursing home or psychiatric hospital. If that is the explicit purpose of the interview, however (e.g., in the context of a suicide threat or attempt), then be clear about it and why. If that is an unlikely outcome, it helps to let the older adult know that you hope to understand her situation and concerns more clearly so you can learn how to help her most appropriately. You can explain that, depending on the circumstances, medications, psychotherapy, group support, home services, or some combination might be recommended.
- *Tell the older adult that you will need to obtain a lot of information during this first interview.* Apologize ahead of time for the fact that you may need to interrupt and redirect questions.
- *Provide the older patient with ample time to respond.* Some elders, especially those who are very depressed or cognitively impaired, will process your questions and formulate their responses slowly. Avoid the temptation to speak for them, or to defer questions to a family member who responds faster. (Eager family members who jump in to answer questions can

be told, "I'd like to hear your father's response first, and *then* I'd like to hear what you have to say.")

- *Be sensitive to your own discomforts.* Do not avoid vital topics that make you feel uncomfortable asking of an older adult (e.g., sexuality, use of alcohol or drugs, issues of disability and dying). Use a matter-of-fact tone and be aware that clinicians are often more uncomfortable about such issues than are their older clients.
- *Encourage questions or challenges to your understanding of things.* Remember that many adults now in their seventies or eighties defer to professionals and may be reluctant to ask questions of the interviewer. Use basic reflection techniques to make sure you have understood the person and give the older adult a chance to correct you.
- *Be aware of the need for privacy and confidentiality.* In some settings (e.g., medical hospital or nursing home), finding a space for an interview out of earshot of roommates or staff can be a challenge requiring cooperation with nursing staff.
- *Know the limits of your competence.* A comprehensive assessment of an older adult with possible depression is often a collaborative effort. In most cases, you will want to obtain the older adult's permission to consult with her medical doctor to be sure that any medical or pharmacological contributions to depression have been ruled out. If you are not a medical professional, you will need to learn about common medical conditions and medications used by older adults. If you have little training in geriatric cognitive assessment, you will need to learn when to refer an older individual with evidence of cognitive difficulties for more extensive neurological or neuropsychological evaluation.

Content/Structure of the Evaluation

The initial clinical interview consists of a standard biopsychosocial history and mental status exam (Silver and Herrmann, 1991). Both details of the individual's personal, medical, and psychiatric history and observations about their behavior are important parts of the evaluation.

Here, we highlight several issues to keep in mind when collecting information during a clinical interview with an older patient. For an excellent overview of "the first session with seniors," see Scogin (2000).

Depending on the referral source and treatment setting, the interviewer may have access to medical or psychiatric records to review before the initial meeting. Or, patients can be asked to bring any records they have (or contact names/numbers of physicians and list of medications they are taking) to the first meeting. Given the complex medical histories of some older patients, this is an efficient way to prepare for the interview. In some practices, it is also possible to have patients complete questionnaires regarding family and psychiatric history, and psychiatric symptoms, prior to the initial meeting, either by mailing materials prior to an outpatient appointment or having individuals arrive early to complete some paperwork.

If it is clear from the referral, or from initial contact with the patient, that the elder is too cognitively or emotionally impaired to provide a reliable history, ask the elder if a family member–or other reliable informant–can be included in the interview. Obtaining optimally reliable information about the course of the illness and prior functioning is critical for determining a diagnostic impression. It is always helpful to ask the older patient, even if others will be interviewed, what her primary concern is or why she believes the referral was made. It is essential to include the elder's perspective to the extent that is possible. Also, do not assume that the informant's report is entirely reliable. For example, caregivers who are depressed have been found to overestimate the extent of depression in the older person for whom they are caring.

As in any psychiatric interview, components of the history will include information about: the onset, course, symptoms, and functional impact of the current problem; any prior psychiatric illness or treatment; current or prior substance abuse; medical and surgical history; family psychiatric history; prescribed and over-the-counter medications being taken; early developmental history, including place and circumstances of birth, family of origin, early illness or trauma, years of school, and early peer relations; occupational history, including military service, jobs, and retirement; social history, including marriage, children, social supports, religious/spiritual practice or belief, financial status, personal interests, and experiences of loss or trauma.

For an adult with 80 years of living, this can be a lot of history to cover. With clinical experience, the interviewer learns to prioritize questions to areas of most critical relevance for the particular case. The interviewer can also include structured assessment tools as indicated to help with the evaluation. For example, the Hamilton Depression Rating Scale (Williams, 1988) can help guide interview-based assessment of depressive symptoms. Or, if grief, anxiety, or alcohol abuse are prominent issues, scales can be administered to help assess these conditions (see Appendix B).

The mental status exam entails the interviewer's observations of the patient's appearance, behavior, speech, affect, thought content, thought process, perception, attention and memory, and insight and judgment. We can learn a lot about a person simply by observing how they present themselves (hygiene? grooming? way of dressing?), communicate (can they see and hear? engage comfortably in discussion?), and respond to questions (with direct and appropriate answers? with rambling stories? with guarded distrust?).

The cognitive evaluation is particularly important in work with older adults, given the relatively high prevalence of memory or other cognitive difficulties. In addition to general behavioral observations, a cognitive screening should be conducted with older patients to assess their orientation (e.g., do they know where they are? the month, date, and year?), concentration, short-term memory, language comprehension and naming, visual-spatial ability, and abstraction skills. Structured cognitive screening tools such as the Mini-Mental State Exam (MMSE) (Folstein, Folstein, and McHugh, 1975) or Modified Mini-Mental State Exam (3MS) (Teng and Chui, 1987) are useful to include in the evaluation (see Appendix B).

Risk assessment is a critical component of any psychiatric evaluation. With older adults, it is important to assess suicidal thoughts, intent, or plan, as well as any history of suicidal behavior or attempt (McIntosh et al., 1994)(see Chapter 7). Other aspects of psychiatric risk include impulse control, aggressiveness, and thoughts of hurting others, as well as extent of insight and judgment about one's problems and potential risks of various behaviors.

For older adults with severe depression and/or dementia, risk assessment must include consideration of the elder's ability to care for herself independently if she is living in the community (Loewenstein and Mogosky, 1999). Obtain information about how much help she needs, if any, with activities of daily living (ADLs: toileting, feeding, dressing, grooming, walking, bathing) and instrumental activities of daily living (IADLs: using the telephone, shopping, preparing food, housekeeping, doing laundry, traveling, managing medications, handling finances) (Lawton, 1971; Lawton and Brody, 1969). Have there been threats to her safety at home, including falls, overuse or underuse of important medications, inadequate nutrition, wandering, motor vehicle accidents, or fires while cooking?

The initial evaluation should yield a general impression of the individual's psychiatric diagnosis. It should produce a sense of the individual's strengths and weaknesses (e.g., relevant to cognition, intelligence, personality features, social supports, history of positive or negative coping) and an appraisal of the impact of current problems on the patient's level of functioning.

With this impression, you are ready to conceive an initial treatment plan, which may be modified over time as you gather further information.

Treatment: General Guidelines and Repertoire of Interventions

Treatment of depression in an older person often entails a combination of interventions. In addition to standard mental health interventions such as antidepressant medication and psychotherapy, it requires a professional stance open to role flexibility, care coordination, interprofessional communication, and advocacy. When devising treatment plans, we value flexibility, pragmatism, and attention to empirically validated interventions. Here we highlight general guidelines for planning treatment with a depressed older adult.

- *Coordinate medical and mental health care.* Medical conditions and treatments often influence psychiatric symptomatology, and elders are at risk for negative medication interactions, particularly when multiple physicians are prescribing. We must know what medications our clients take and why. Mental health professionals must routinely obtain release of information forms to obtain medical history from treating physicians. Likewise, medical care providers may need to be informed about the impact of psychiatric illness on the patient's functioning.

- *Become comfortable with role flexibility.* Due to the multiple needs of complex geriatric patients, most care providers find themselves stretched to the limits of their professional roles. In some instances, home visits may be called for by professionals who have not been trained to offer treatment outside their offices (e.g., psychologists). More active outreach, case management, and care coordination—all accomplished with respect for the older individual's right to confidentiality and informed consent—are also often necessary.
- *Provide psychoeducation.* Educate older adults about depression and the goals and process of mental health interventions that may be new to them. Do not assume that the older adult, or the family, knows "how to be in therapy." Instead, take a relatively active stance in providing structure, information, and summaries of what has been covered in treatment sessions.
- *Recognize the effectiveness of psychotherapy.* Depressed older adults benefit from psychotherapy in individual, group, or family contexts (Karel and Hinrichsen, 2000; Scogin and McElreath, 1994). To date, cognitive-behavioral and interpersonal therapies have received the most empirical support as effective treatments for this population.
    - *Cognitive-behavioral psychotherapy (CBT)* (Coon et al., 1999; Gallagher-Thompson and Thompson, 1996; Zeiss and Steffen, 1996). Behavioral and cognitive therapy approaches are empirically validated treatments for depression in adults (Chambliss et al., 1996). Behavior therapy focuses on the relationship between activity and mood, and encourages increased participation in pleasant activities, decreased participation in aversive activities, and improved problem-solving and social skills. Cognitive therapy focuses on the relationship between distorted thinking and negative

moods and behaviors, and helps the depressed patient to identify, challenge, and replace depressive thoughts with more realistic thoughts. Often, cognitive and behavioral strategies are used together (CBT). These active, collaborative, goal-focused treatments are easily adapted to work with older adults. CBT has been shown to help older adults recover from and prevent relapse of depression.

- *Interpersonal psychotherapy (IPT)* (Hinrichsen, 1999; Klerman et al., 1984; Reynolds et al., 1999; Weissman, Markowitz, and Klerman, 2000). IPT is also an empirically validated treatment for depression in adults (Chambliss et al., 1996), and is based on understanding depression as both affecting and being affected by interpersonal relationships. It is a collaborative, goal-focused psychotherapy that aims to address one (or two) of four interpersonal problem areas: grief (death of a loved one), interpersonal disputes (conflict with significant others), role transition (change in life circumstances, e.g., retirement), and deficits in interpersonal skills. The prevalence of these themes in the lives of many elders makes IPT appealing at face value. It, too, has been shown to help older adults recover from and prevent relapse of depression.
- *Other modalities.* Although there is little to no research to date supporting the use of other psychotherapies with depressed older adults, clinical experience and the literature suggest that depressed older adults may also benefit from psychodynamic (Lazarus, 1988; Nemiroff and Colarusso, 1985), family (Hinrichsen and Zweig, 1994), existential (Brody, 1999), and a variety of group (Kemp, Corgiat, and Gill, 1992; Leszcz, 1990; Sprenkel, 1999) interventions.

- *Know about safe and effective psychopharmacological interventions.* Too often, depressed older adults are treated with inappropriate classes or dosages of psychotropic medication. They can benefit from antidepressant medications (McCusker et al., 1998); in cases of moderate to severe depression, a combination of medication and psychotherapy has been shown to have the best outcomes. Communication and attention to systemic context are critical to medication effectiveness since an older adult with visual deficits and cognitive decline, for instance, cannot be expected to remember to take his medication or to be able to read the instructions on the bottle. (See Appendix A for a psychopharmacology overview.)

- *Treat major depression as a chronic, recurring illness.* Depression frequently relapses in older adults who are not monitored and treated as needed over time. Older adults with major depression benefit from "maintenance" medication and psychotherapy after remission of the depressive episode (Reynolds, 1997). Build follow-ups after acute treatment into your treatment plan.
- *Know when to consider ECT.* Electroconvulsive therapy (ECT) is an important treatment for major depression in some older adults. It should be considered when the depression is life-threatening, when the patient has a severe depression with psychotic features, when a rapid response is vital (e.g., the patient is not eating), or when medications cannot be tolerated or have failed to produce a response (Kelly and Zisselman, 2000; Sackeim, 1994).
- *Monitor treatment response.* Continue to monitor the patient's level of depression as well as his response to specific treatment goals (e.g., targeted amounts of sleep, exercise, social outings). Improved scores on a depression scale (e.g., the Beck Depression Inventory) can be a source of hope to the patient that treatment is helping, whereas evidence of no change or worsening depression suggests that we need to reevaluate our interventions (e.g., raise dosage or change altogether an antidepressant medication).
- *Refer to a specialist when needed.* In complex cases, you may need consultation and/or collaboration with another professional–a psychiatrist, specialty medical provider, psychologist, neuropsychologist, social worker, nurse, case manager, physical therapist, speech therapist, nutritionist, occupational therapist, pharmacist, or chaplain.

- *Know about your local referral network and service agencies.* Find out about your local Area Agency on Aging (see Appendix D, Administration on Aging Web site), and what services are available for which seniors meeting what criteria (income, disability, homebound status). Be aware of the informal support network of the seniors you serve (e.g., do they have access to rides to appointments?).
- *Learn about the continuum of care in your community.* Older adults treated for depression may require a range of care in a range of settings, including acute psychiatric inpatient care, psychiatric day hospital, outpatient mental health, adult day care, ambulatory and inpatient medical services, and home care services.
- *Learn about Medicare and other insurance.* Become aware of reimbursement issues for mental health services, particularly Medicare policies in your area. Limits to coverage will affect the ability of many elders to afford mental health services. (At present, basic Medicare does *not* cover prescription drug benefits.) See the readings and Web sites listed in Appendix D.
- *Be innovative.* A lot of room exists for improving the quality and systems of care to older adults with mental health concerns (Hartman-Stein, 1998). Become aware of care models receiving research attention and validation. Create and be on the lookout for opportunities to institute such models, such as the example of mental health professionals establishing liaisons with primary care practices that serve older adults. See Appendix C for other examples of innovative care models.

With this repertoire of possible therapies, and an awareness of resources for care coordination, you are able to target interventions to the needs of the particular older adult. In Part II, we illustrate how these strategies for intervening with depressed elders can be applied in a range of individual cases.

PART TWO

Cases

The following fourteen case studies illustrate a range of diagnostic issues, medical and psychosocial problems, care settings, and treatment approaches encountered in working with depressed older adults. They are all based on our own clinical work and typically represent a synthesis of several patients' experiences. In every instance, we altered names, places, details of personal history, and certain aspects of care to protect confidentiality.

We chose to present cases that had relatively positive outcomes, albeit to varying degrees, because our goal was to provide models of how interventions can help when they are successful. Sometimes "help" does not entail "cure," but rather preventing increased severity of depression or optimizing functioning in the context of multiple chronic problems.

For illustrative purposes, we describe a disproportionate number of severe depressions; the cases selected are not intended to represent the distribution of types that end up in treatment. In fact, the majority of older adults treated for depression are seen in primary care settings where they receive antidepressant medications. In our case studies, however, all patients have received specialty mental health care.

Finally, we focus the case descriptions on clinical assessment and treatment issues and do not explicitly address how services were paid for. Obviously, this is a vital issue and each situation differs, depending on the individual's income, insurance coverage, site of care, and state of residence. In general, Medicare is the primary health insurance for older adults and, as of this writing, efforts are under way to increase its coverage for mental health services. Co-payments are typically paid for out-of-pocket, by supplemental insurance, or by Medicaid. Please see the readings and Web sites listed in Appendix D for more information on funding for mental health services.

CHAPTER FOUR

Minor Depression: Eleanor Peterson

Subsyndromal depressive symptoms are relatively common in late life, and increase with advancing age. Adults in their seventies, eighties, and beyond are more and more likely to suffer disabling physical, sensory, and/or cognitive conditions that affect their ability to function as they once did; this functional disability is strongly associated with minor depression (Beekman et al., 1995; Koenig and Blazer, 1996). Eleanor's case highlights the issue of vision loss in late life, and how such loss can put someone at risk for depression.

Both vision and hearing loss are increasingly common in later years, and can lead to declines in activity, social isolation, and restrictions to one's independence. Assistive devices and other rehabilitation programs can help older adults adapt to sensory loss. However, minor depression in reaction to such losses can lead to excess disability, whereby an individual loses motivation or hope to do the work it takes to optimize her functioning. Eleanor's depression put her at risk for less-than-optimal adaptation to her failing vision. A group therapy intervention helped her (Finkel, 1991; Kemp, Corgiat, and Gill, 1992; Leszcz, 1990; Sprenkel, 1999).

Eleanor Peterson: Introduction

Eleanor was a 92-year-old, twice widowed, retired elementary education teacher who had never had children. She prided herself on and felt blessed by her good health. In her late eighties, Eleanor developed macular degeneration. Eventually her vision decreased to the point where she had to stop driving.

Then, she developed cataracts in both eyes. With ongoing difficulties preparing her own meals and managing other household chores, she decided to move into an assisted living facility serving adults with vision loss. She missed her home and her ability to read and do other usual activities, and at times felt sad and anxious about her future. For the most part, however, she was able to enjoy living and sharing activities with other partially sighted people for the two years she lived at the facility.

One year ago, she had successful cataract surgery on her left eye. However, complications of the same surgery on the right eye several months later caused permanent blindness in that one. Meanwhile, the vision in her left eye continued to deteriorate from the macular degeneration, and she began to worry that she would become functionally blind. She started to feel worthless and tearful, could not concentrate as well on her books-on-tape, and was spending more time alone in her room. An occupational therapist at the facility noted that Eleanor did not seem to be her upbeat self—she appeared sad, tired, and was isolating herself from her usual friends and activities—and, after speaking with Eleanor, asked if she would be willing to go for an evaluation at the local psychiatric outpatient clinic, which had a range of geriatric services. Eleanor agreed to the referral.

Issues for Consideration

Losing the ability to see is a difficult loss. What can help someone come to terms with such a loss? It depends, in part, on its particular meaning for that person. For Eleanor, what about losing her vision made her feel particularly frightened or hopeless? Was it her ability to do certain things for herself, a fear of increased vulnerability, or something else? What has helped her cope with prior losses and challenges in her life?

Professionals working with older adults in residential, community, or clinical settings need to be alert for signs of depression in their clients. Eleanor, who did not identify the signs in herself, was fortunate to have captured the interest of the local occupational therapist, who recognized them and encouraged the mental health referral.

Assessment

Eleanor completed an intake interview with the clinic social worker and had no difficulty answering questions about her life and her current concerns. The social worker observed that, in walking from the waiting room to her office, Eleanor ambulated as easily as a 75-year-old. She was petite and thin but healthy-appearing and carefully groomed; she carried herself with comfort and dignity. Eleanor explained that she had always been very healthy, active, and happy. She prided herself on never needing medication her entire life, except for the one aspirin she took when her mother died.

She spoke of grieving the losses of both her husbands, thirty and fifteen years earlier, but over the years had maintained many friendships and interests, including gardening, classical music, reading, crosswords, and volunteering for local political candidates. At the age of 92, she had survived most of her friends but had made new ones at the assisted living facility. While having to give up reading and other interests, she had started to listen to books-on-tape, do crosswords with the help of a college volunteer, and listen to news radio.

The social worker asked Eleanor to talk about her vision loss. Eleanor explained that she could see out of the periphery of her left eye, allowing her to negotiate her way around the building and recognize people she knew. She tearfully spoke of her fear of becoming one of the most visually impaired people at the facility, afraid that her partially sighted peers would reject her if she became totally blind. Although she knew from the ophthalmologist that she would maintain some peripheral vision, she could not help fearing that her left eye would go blind as her right one did. Having always coped with her vision loss by reminding herself that others were worse off than she, she now feared she'd be the worst off.

Eleanor admitted to the social worker that, for the past six months or so, she had been feeling rejected by her peers and was isolating herself. She described feeling sad about her future, feeling worthless, and having occasional trouble staying asleep at night. She also said she worried that she might be getting Alzheimer's disease, because she felt her memory was slipping and she just couldn't focus on things like she used to. She scored 14 out of 30 points on the Geriatric Depression Scale, suggesting a moderate degree of depression, but she did not report problems with appetite, psychomotor slowing or agitation, loss of capacity for pleasure, or thoughts of death. On the cognitive screen, she scored 28 of 28 points on the MMSE (excluding two vision-dependent items).

Eleanor was relieved when told that the screening, together with her ability to communicate a clear and coherent history, showed that she was not "losing her faculties." The social worker explained that depression can affect one's concentration and this was the likely cause of Eleanor's perceived memory trouble. Although somewhat skeptical about mental health treatment, Eleanor was willing to consider that the group therapy the social worker recommended might indeed help her.

Conceptualization

Eleanor had a long history of good health and positive coping. When her usual coping resources were overwhelmed by the threat of blindness, she evidenced depressive symptoms affecting her ability to function. She was isolating herself and thus feeling more rejected, and was not keeping up with the usual activities that helped her enjoy life and feel good about herself.

Though she did not meet criteria for major depression, her changes in mood, sleep, and hopefulness, and their impact on her functioning, could be conceptualized as a minor depression. As these symptoms and related functional disability have persisted for more than six months beyond the initial adjustment to her surgical complications, intervention is warranted. Of note, Eleanor's concern about her memory functioning is a common sign of depression in older adults, who—fearing onset of dementia—can be vigilant about their cognition; the concentration difficulties common to depression exacerbate these fears.

Having assessed Eleanor's need for support in coping with disability, increased social isolation, and feared rejection by peers, the social worker suggested that Eleanor join a group psychotherapy program for older adults whose physical and/or interpersonal losses, like hers, had precipitated mood disorders. Eleanor's intact cognitive capacity, verbal ability, and good hearing, as well as the fact that her facility offered transportation to the sessions, made her an ideal candidate for group treatment.

Treatment

Eleanor participated in an outpatient group therapy program, which met twice weekly for five weeks. The group focused on both sharing feelings of loss and supporting members in strategies to focus on activities and relationships for which they remained able to engage. The group included seven older men and women, among them a 68-year-old man completely paralyzed on one side of his body by a stroke and a woman who had lived 55 of her 75 years in the grip of a terrible marriage. Their stories reminded Eleanor of her good physical health and her positive relationships with both husbands; she thanked God that she was 92 years old and still going strong.

In the group context, Eleanor was able to reactivate the coping style that had been so adaptive until it was overwhelmed by her loss of sight: When she recognized and compared herself to people even worse off than she, her appreciation for what she had transcended her disappointment over what she had lost. She found that she was able to help other members of the group by encouraging them too to focus on their strengths. The group's positive feedback prompted her to risk extending herself again to friends at the assisted living facility, and she discovered that they were actually quite receptive to her efforts. She hadn't considered that her self-isolating behavior might have actually pushed her friends away.

Eleanor also made an effort to reengage with some positive activities. She decided to buy a better tape recorder for her books-on-tape and classical cassettes. She started walking regularly and began a T'ai Chi class at the local senior center. As she gradually became better able to sleep and less anxious about her future, she regained her capacity to make the most of the resources she had.

Comment

Older adults facing what would seem to be devastating disabilities, and experiencing depressive reactions, can adapt and find renewed motivation and hope, particularly those with a long history of positive coping. Most people who reach very old age have a lifetime of coping resources upon which to draw. (Indeed, the fact that the majority do not become depressed with advancing frailty speaks to the amazing resilience and adaptability of the human spirit.) Certainly, adaptation becomes more difficult with decreasing physical or cognitive reserves, particularly when coupled with potential loss of important social supports.

This case illustrates that one can't be "too old" to benefit from psychotherapeutic interventions. In particular, group interventions can meet the needs of older adults struggling with disability and depression. Participating in groups makes people feel less alone and supplies a forum in which they can identify or recover positive coping strategies; the real opportunity to help one another also contributes to a renewed sense of meaning and self-worth.

CHAPTER FIVE

Complicated Grief and Depression: Pauline Feld

One of the costs of living a long life is surviving many of one's family and friends. Because women tend to outlive men, the majority of older women who were married become widowed as they survive past the age of 65. With increasing age, people are also more likely to face the loss of siblings, lifelong friends, and adult children. Most older adults grieve normally, consistent with their cultural background and surviving support systems, and are able to adjust to the loss and construct a life without the loved one. Such loss, however, does put older adults at increased risk for major depression, complicated grief reactions, or both. Pauline's case illustrates how a mental health intervention can help a bereaved older adult cope with a loss and recover from associated depression or complicated grief reactions.

Pauline Feld: Introduction

> Pauline Feld was a 73-year-old Jewish woman who had been happily married for 48 years when her husband Joseph died suddenly from a heart attack. Almost two years after his death, her grief was still interrupting her appetite and concentration; she continued to think of Joe all the time and to blame herself for his death. Pauline could not understand this enduring grief, as she had managed to survive the death of her daughter Sharon ten years earlier. The Trazodone prescribed by her primary care doctor last year was helping her sleep, but her grief continued. Her doctor now referred her to a local mental health practice for psychotherapy. She had previously refused to join

the widow support group at the synagogue, believing it would be too upsetting to hear of others' losses and not wanting to burden others with her own. She agreed to the individual psychotherapy referral.

Issues for Consideration

While most older adults are not new to loss, it is important to understand the person's particular history of loss and grief over their lifetime. Cumulative losses can affect a person's experience of grief. Pauline had experienced at least one previous significant loss, the death of her daughter. How has she coped with that and other losses? What personal and interpersonal strengths and vulnerabilities does she have that affect her adaptation to loss? Understanding the particular loss is also important. How did Pauline and her husband relate to each other and what particular voids did his absence create for her?

Clarifying Pauline's diagnostic presentation is also important. After a loss, most people experience normal bereavement reactions that do not develop into major depression. Some people experience complicated grief, however, which embodies elements of posttraumatic stress (feelings of disbelief and being stunned) and separation distress (preoccupation with thoughts of the deceased, yearning, searching) (Prigerson et al., 1995a). Complicated grief is distinct from, and can be more enduring than, depression, with which it may or may not be concurrent; it is potentially functionally disabling, and does not appear to be helped by antidepressant medication (Rosenzweig et al., 1997; Thompson et al., 1991). Is Pauline suffering from complicated grief, major depression, or both?

Various interventions can help individuals who are grieving. While participating in support groups offered through churches or community centers can be enormously beneficial for normal grievers, psychotherapy is indicated for people with enduring depression or functional disability related to grief. Interpersonal psychotherapy (IPT), a time-limited treatment that focuses on interpersonal issues that appear tied to the onset or maintenance of depression, is particularly well suited for depressed, bereaved elders (Hinrichsen, 1999; Weissman,

Markowitz, and Klerman, 2000). When focused on grief, IPT facilitates the emotional expression of grief and helps with the practical and emotional adjustments to living life without the deceased.

Widowed elders are apt to have to deal with practical matters previously handled by the deceased spouse and with disposition of his possessions; financial, residential, and legal decisions; expanding independent activities and learning to relate to others as an uncoupled individual; ambivalent, perhaps angry, feelings about the death and about the marriage itself; and coping with feelings about prior losses (Miller et al., 1994). The therapist would want to address this range of issues in her evaluation.

Assessment

When Pauline met with the psychologist, she completed questionnaires that measured her level of depression [Beck Depression Inventory (BDI) score of 19, suggesting moderate depression] and her feelings of grief [Inventory of Complicated Grief (ICG) score of 36, suggesting a complicated grief reaction](Prigerson et al., 1995b). A brief cognitive screen showed no signs of memory or other cognitive problems (MMSE = 30/30). Having recently seen her primary care doctor, Pauline was able to confirm that her physical health was stable. Answering many questions about her life and relationships during the course of the interview, she was variously tearful, funny, self-deprecating, and apologetic for her moments of "weakness."

Pauline and Joe had retired five years prior to Joe's death, she from part-time work in the local library and he from his own printing business. Joe was always a steady, reliable provider, and a gentle and shy man who relied on Pauline to plan their family and other social activities. They had raised three daughters and a son, and the whole family grieved when their middle daughter, Sharon, died from breast cancer at the age of 38, some ten years earlier. Sharon had a strong and capable husband (David) and two adolescent boys who survived her; the entire family came together to help the boys through some difficult years. All the children and grandchildren lived within one hour's drive and they got together frequently.

When Sharon died, Pauline had difficulty accepting that the doctors could not save her and was angry at the injustice that she should have survived one of her children. During the next year, she divided her time between the library and keeping the household going for David and the boys, firmly determined to remain strong for them—and also for her husband, who, she knew, couldn't stand to see her cry. Joe was more religious than she, and he seemed to derive comfort from his faith and weekly recitation of the mourner's prayer at the synagogue. After a few years, the family was getting used to Sharon's absence and, although anniversaries, birthdays, and holidays continued to be sad without her, everyone was busy and doing relatively well.

Pauline was not new to helping the family through difficult times. Her father had died of cancer when she was a teenager; at the time, her two older brothers were already married and out of the home. Pauline's mother, Bessie, was very depressed and, while Pauline's brothers were able to offer some financial assistance, Pauline took much of the responsibility for caring for herself and her mother at home. Years later, when Bessie suffered a stroke, Pauline and Joe took her into their home for several years until her death.

When Pauline and Joe retired, both were in decent health, although Joe, being treated for hypertension, knew he needed to lose some weight, and Pauline was troubled by arthritis in her back. They slowed down a bit and enjoyed themselves with their grandchildren, in their garden, visiting friends on the coast, and just relaxing. One fall day, when Joe was out raking leaves, he had a heart attack and died in the ambulance on the way to the hospital.

Pauline was stunned and overwhelmed. She could not believe he was gone. Over time, she felt that she could go through the motions of her everyday life, but she continued to feel empty and alone and, at times, even felt that she was going crazy. She found herself crying uncontrollably at night when she was alone, which scared her. She did not cry in front of the family, knowing they were upset enough without worrying about her. She saw several girlfriends, but tended to refuse offers to go out with the couples with whom she and Joe had previously socialized. She felt awkward without Joe and was sure they felt awkward too.

In her house, she felt Joe's presence and everything there reminded her of him. She could not help thinking that, if she had made him go to the doctor sooner, or had pushed him to let their grandson rake the leaves, or had been better about cooking healthy foods for him, he would still be here. She could simply not accept that he was gone, and she was ashamed of feeling such continued despair after almost two years. Despite her emotional suffering, when asked, Pauline was clear that she did not want to die nor did she entertain thoughts of suicide; she wanted to enjoy and be of help to her family for whatever time she had left.

On the basis of the evaluation, the psychologist discussed with Pauline that she appeared to be suffering both from major depression and from complicated grief and recommended that they meet for a course of interpersonal psychotherapy—a short-term treatment that could help people who were depressed secondary to grief.

Conceptualization

Pauline did not appear to have medical contributions to her depression, although her activities were limited slightly by arthritic pain. She had a good relationship with and was followed closely by her physician. Psychologically, she had a history of losses, and helping her to identify how she coped with prior and current losses would be important. Socially, she was also facing changes in her roles and relationships, for she was now a noncoupled woman without regular caregiving responsibilities or daily commitments for the first time in many years. Both major depression and complicated grief were making it difficult for her to adapt to these changes.

Pauline's independent and stoic style made her initially uncomfortable with the idea of seeking treatment, of allowing herself to be vulnerable. She had no history of mental health treatment, and the therapist would need to keep in mind what type of generational misconceptions she might have brought to the therapy. She also brought many resources to the treatment, including her intelligence, humor, close relations with surviving adult children, and ability to get along well with others.

Treatment

During the initial phase of treatment the psychologist educated Pauline about depression and grief. The psychologist explained that grief is a normal and expectable response to a loss, but for some the process is much more difficult. The chief difficulty for Pauline was that she now had major depression, a psychiatric illness that was impairing her ability to function. The meaning of her score on the BDI was reviewed with her. The therapist explained that researchers have found that depression in most people can be treated effectively with psychotherapy, medication, or a combination of these, and that she had hope that Pauline would show improvement. This education was very helpful to Pauline; having been afraid of her feelings of despair and vulnerability, she was relieved to learn that her experiences were common syndromes following the death of one's spouse.

During the initial phase of treatment, the therapist also reviewed significant relationships in Pauline's life to determine whether there might be additional interpersonal stresses tied to her depression. There appeared to be none. At this point, the psychologist explained her understanding of Pauline's problem, treatment goals, and how IPT would be conducted over 16 weeks. Pauline said she felt the therapist understood her situation and, although not particularly comfortable receiving help, she agreed to the plan. She was able to see the therapy as something she could do to help herself.

During the middle phase of treatment, the therapist utilized IPT strategies for treating grief: reviewing depressive symptoms and their relationship to the loss; reconstructing Pauline's relationship with her husband; encouraging her to describe the sequence and consequence of events just prior to, during, and after her husband's death; exploring associated negative and positive feelings; and helping Pauline to consider ways of becoming reinvolved with others.

Pauline described in detail what happened the day of her husband's death and the weeks that followed. She said she had discussed this with a few people but was reluctant to burden others with her problems. She wept while discussing the horror of finding her husband unconscious and how she tried to busy herself after his death so that she would not be overwhelmed by feelings of grief.

Discussion of her husband's death quickly led into discussion of her father's death when she was 16, and the immediate pressure she felt to care for others and not to grieve herself. She expressed anger at her mother for her dependence on her when she was just a teenager. And then there was Sharon's death. Why hadn't she forced Sharon to get a mastectomy when the cancer was first diagnosed? Why hadn't God taken her rather than her daughter? When Sharon died, Pauline felt she had lost a piece of herself, but she quickly mobilized to take care of her grandsons. She also found herself providing a lot of support to her husband, who was disconsolate over Sharon's death.

Over the course of several months in therapy, Pauline expressed a range of complicated feelings about the losses in her life and her role as caregiver. She was able to see how caring for others protected her at those times from dealing with her own grief and, now, with her husband gone, she did not have anyone immediately needing her care. She still felt stuck, unable to come to terms with her husband's death. The therapist suggested she bring in pictures of Joe over his lifetime. At first she was reluctant, but then she brought in several family albums. As she paged through the albums she told stories of their early life together, the joys and stresses of raising four children, and problems in their relationship that "I just had to live with." In the process of telling these stories, she frequently wept, laughed, and expressed anger. Midway through the therapy, she began to box up his clothing to send to charity and confided that she drew a special comfort in the touch and smell of his clothing.

Pauline increasingly began to review options for "getting on with life." She began exercising regularly at the local pool (which was good for her arthritis as well as her spirit), renewed acquaintance with some old friends, and joined a women's group at the synagogue.

During the last weeks of psychotherapy, Pauline reported improved appetite and concentration, interest in social and other activities, and less sense of self-blame and worthlessness; she was pleased to see that her BDI and ICG scores had declined significantly (scores of 8 and 16, respectively). Pauline thanked the therapist for all her help; the therapist told Pauline that her gains resulted from her active involvement in therapy, her willingness to explore options, and her work to refashion a new life. Pauline was nervous that ending treatment might lead to a return of depression. The therapist assured Pauline that this was a common fear and she felt confident that Pauline would do well. Nonetheless, Pauline requested, and the therapist agreed to, several monthly sessions.

Pauline saw the therapist two more times, during which the gains she had made were reinforced. At this time, Pauline also saw her primary care doctor and asked if she could taper off the Trazodone. She did this and her sleep remained fine. Pauline told the therapist that she felt she could "do things on my own now" and ended their visits.

Comment

Pauline had not previously allowed herself to grieve; rather, she had worked very hard to remain "strong" for others in the family. Therapy provided her with permission to process her grief experience; a relationship with an empathic therapist helped her to explore how her reaction to previous losses might have affected her ability to cope with her husband's sudden death. Psychotherapy helped her depression to remit.

Pauline had personal and interpersonal resources that some bereaved elders do not. Working with elders who are socially isolated presents special challenges, especially for those whose spouse may have been their only close support. Often, older men have limited social networks apart from those established by their wives. In these cases, helping the older adult to expand sources of support (e.g., taking meals at a senior lunch program to promote social contact, if desired) is important. When a frail older adult loses a spouse or other important caregiver, alternative care and residential options often need to be explored. Finally, bereaved older adults are at risk for increased morbidity and mortality, including suicide risk; outreach and risk assessment with these elders are important (Cummings, 1998).

CHAPTER SIX

Dysthymia: Theresa Sanchez

Dysthymia, a chronic depression less severe than major depressive disorder, is not an uncommon diagnosis among older adults with depressive symptoms. Some experience it for the first time in later years, whereas others carry long-standing dysthymic symptoms into their old age. To what extent dysthymia in late life may reflect underlying brain changes, chronic adjustment disorders with depressive features, or something else remains open to continued research. In this case, Theresa experienced chronic depressive symptoms as she had increased difficulty dealing with long-standing marital conflict and was learning to handle pain in her hip. Cognitive-behavioral psychotherapy helped her to improve her coping strategies, to reduce depressive symptoms, and to increase her sense of self-worth.

Theresa Sanchez: Introduction

Theresa was a 74-year-old Mexican-American woman who was financially dependent on her husband, Peter. She'd had a miserable marriage, almost from the beginning. She and Peter had both wanted out of their parents' homes, and getting married had seemed convenient. But after years of trying to have kids, and discovering that they could not do so, the blaming, finger-pointing, and arguing between them got worse. For years, Theresa relied on the support of her sister Inez and spent much of her time with Inez and her children. But then Inez moved across the state following her stroke two years ago to be closer to her daughter. Now Theresa spent most of her time at home, watching TV, snacking, cleaning, and preparing dinner for when Peter arrived home late in the afternoon. A gruff and unhappy man, Peter had never allowed Theresa to work outside of the home, and he did pay the bills. Although he never physically hurt her, he always yelled at and criticized her. She didn't see a way out.

In addition to her loneliness and chronic marital strain, Theresa had developed severe pain in her hip over the past few months. After she finally got up the courage to tell Peter and to see a doctor, she was diagnosed with a sciatic nerve problem. She attended two sessions of physical therapy, and was relieved to learn that, if she did the exercises prescribed by the physical therapist twice a day, she was able to manage the pain. But she still felt nervous, sad, lonely, and hopeless about her future, and she was eating too much and upset that she was gaining weight.

Years ago Theresa heard her niece talking about counseling, and thought something like that might help her, but she never thought she could afford it. When she heard a radio ad offering free counseling for depressed people who wanted to participate in a research program, she took note of it, even though she really didn't think she was "mental."

Issues for Consideration

Older adults may not know how to find mental health services, even if they want to consider using them. Outreach programs that can normalize their use as accessible, affordable, and potentially helpful, like the radio advertisement that caught Theresa's interest, are important for reaching older adults.

The interacting influence of cohort, gender, ethnicity, religion, and individual factors is always important to remember. These factors affect people's openness to the idea of mental health services, as well as their basic values and beliefs about life and relationships. Getting to know the person in these contexts is, of course, always a part of the work. As for Theresa specifically, what generational, cultural, and/or gender issues may affect her adaptation and be relevant for her care? What is it like for an older Latina to turn for help outside the family, and not to have her own children to rely on for help in later years? Given the dominance of her husband in their traditional Hispanic household, what options would Theresa be willing to consider to help herself (Haley, Han, and Henderson, 1998; Morales, 1999)?

Assessment

When Theresa called the number announced on the radio, she was surprised to be offered an interview later that week and was able to catch the bus to the clinic. She met with a female psychologist who asked her many questions about her life and background. The psychologist observed Theresa to be overweight and neatly groomed, wearing a simple dress and sandals, and to have no difficulty walking, seeing, or hearing; she did use glasses to read. Though Theresa initially seemed a bit shy, she was easily engaged and, over the course of the interview, "spilled" her story, sometimes with tears and sometimes with laughter. She spoke English fluently, although she and Peter used mostly Spanish at home, and appeared relieved to talk to a kind woman about her troubles.

Theresa discussed her depriving experience growing up as the fifth of eight children. Her father drank excessively, and was physically and verbally abusive to her mother. She married Peter when she was young to get away from her parents and so many siblings. Although she and Inez, her next oldest sister, remained close, she maintained little contact with her other siblings. She thought if she and Peter could just have a few children of their own, her life would settle down. But when the doctors said they each had a fertility problem, it was quite a blow. The only real identity for which Theresa was prepared was that of a wife and mother. She and Peter fought for years.

Theresa remained involved with the church, and while she went to Mass every Sunday, she missed sharing it with Inez since her move. Years ago, she had tried to talk to the priest about her difficult marriage; however, when he questioned her commitment to her husband, she just felt more discouraged. Since then, she did not often confide in him.

For years Theresa felt a sense of isolation, sadness, self-doubt, and "nerves." Lately, she was having trouble sleeping, was crying more often, was lonely, bored, and restless; she didn't know where to turn. During the assessment, she completed the Beck Depression Inventory and scored in the moderately depressed range (BDI = 18). She evidenced no cognitive difficulties on a brief screening (MMSE = 28/30). A report of her recent medical exam—obtained with Theresa's consent from her primary care doctor—documented that she was mildly overweight with high cholesterol, had arthritis in her hands, and suffered hip pain from her sciatica. She took Tylenol for her arthritis and was advised to watch her diet and walk more regularly. Though she knew she was eating too much and not walking enough, she was committed to doing her physical therapy exercises for the sciatica. She denied suicidal thoughts, or any history of suicidal thinking, and took good care of her hygiene, grooming, and household responsibilities. She did not meet full diagnostic criteria for major depression but did meet criteria for dysthymia. She was interested to try a course of individual psychotherapy.

Conceptualization

Theresa had multiple chronic stressors contributing to her depressive symptoms. She did not appear to require further medical or neurological workup. The loss of her sister's support and companionship, combined with her finding herself more limited physically, complicated Theresa's long-standing sense of loss and unworthiness in a difficult marriage without the children she had hoped for. Theresa's strengths included her faith and commitment to her values, her pride in taking care of herself and her home, and her capacity for humor and relating well to people. She appeared to be an excellent candidate for the cognitive-behavioral therapy program, as she was motivated for treatment and had demonstrated through her physical therapy progress that she could collaborate and take responsibility for helping herself feel better.

As in all treatment planning, it would be important for Theresa and the therapist to define treatment objectives consistent with

Theresa's values and beliefs. For example, certain objectives (e.g., leaving her husband or getting a job) proved unrealistic for Theresa once discussed. Realistic treatment goals could include helping her to engage in more pleasant activities for herself, expand her social network, increase her assertiveness skills, and understand and alter her negative thought patterns.

Treatment

Theresa was assigned to a twelve-week course of weekly individual cognitive-behavioral psychotherapy for depression, with 4 booster sessions at one-month intervals after weekly treatment was completed. The therapy focused on: mood monitoring; identifying and increasing pleasant activities (particularly social activities); increasing assertiveness skills; and completing daily thought records to understand her negative thought patterns (Gallagher-Thompson and Thompson, 1996).

Initially, Theresa chiefly blamed her husband for her current mood. Her thought records indicated that she viewed him as verbally abusive, demeaning, and controlling. She said that she stayed with him because of financial necessity as well as her commitment to her marital vows. Daily mood monitoring confirmed that her mood was strongly related to thoughts about and interactions with Peter, and she commented that she had been socialized to focus on her husband's needs and well-being. To imagine that perhaps, at this stage of her life, she could allow herself to address some of her own wants and likes represented quite a change. After she identified that she would enjoy being around other people more often, she began attending free lunches at the local senior center, where she met another woman who attended her church. Together, they decided to volunteer in the church's meals program for the homeless.

The therapy helped to challenge Theresa's core beliefs that she was defective and flawed, beliefs she had held particularly since her infertility problems and that Peter's history of criticizing her had reinforced. Together, she and the therapist worked to examine actual situations in which Theresa believed she was defective—and to evaluate this belief from a more rational perspective and consider alternative explanations. Over time, Theresa could see that, while she was not perfect, her infertility and Peter's unhappiness with his life did not make her defective.

Theresa's mood improved as she spent more time out of the house with people and tested new ways to look at herself and her situation. She saw that her BDI score, which was monitored each week, was declining and she tended to attribute the improvement to the therapist's direct guidance or simply to having had an "easier" week. The therapist encouraged Theresa to consider how she, herself, was contributing to the change: "You know Theresa, in reality, your situation this week is no different than it was last week. But, YOU are different. You are looking at the world a different way, doing things that you enjoy, and taking care of yourself." And when the therapist asked again the following week how she understood her improved mood, Theresa responded, "You asked me this last week, and you were right—my situation [living with husband] had not changed at all—but I have changed—I realized it must be something different about me, something different I'm doing. All week long that has given me hope to get better."

At the end of twelve weeks of individual treatment, Theresa was beginning to be aware of her own needs and taking steps to meet them. Her increased time with a new friend and volunteering helped her to feel valued, while her decreased time snacking in front of the TV helped her to lose a few pounds. Her husband did not interfere, as long as she continued to prepare their evening meal, which she was committed to do. By the end of the treatment, four months later, Theresa no longer met criteria for dysthymia. Though she remained sad but accepting of her unsatisfying marriage, she was learning to be less reactive to Peter's moods. And, with new skills to manage her activities and her thoughts, she was feeling better about herself.

Comment

Cognitive-behavioral therapy is known as an effective treatment for depression and is easily adapted to work with older adults. For elders who are feeling a loss of control over their health, relationships, or other life circumstances, an intervention that teaches how mood can be affected by thoughts and behaviors can lead to an increased sense of control and self-efficacy. As to the efficacy of psychotherapy for dysthymia, particularly in older adults, research remains limited and in fact one recent study found that antidepressant medication (paroxetine) was more effective in this context than problem-solving psychotherapy (Williams et al., 2000). Had Theresa not had a positive response to the psychotherapy, she would have been offered psychiatric consultation to consider an antidepressant medication. But because of her ease in forming a collaborative relationship with her therapist and her motivation and willingness to try new things, she turned out to be a great psychotherapy candidate.

In working with ethnic elders, interventions that focus on problems and solutions are more likely to be accepted than insight-oriented therapies (Morales, 1999). For many older women who were socialized to primary roles as caregivers to husbands, children, or parents, focusing on one's own needs and desires is a new and possibly disorienting experience. Therapists working with older adults must be sensitive to and respectful of generational and cultural beliefs that may not be open to modification, while remaining on the lookout for areas of openness to try something new.

CHAPTER SEVEN

Suicidal Depression: Samuel Schmitt

Most older adults who commit suicide are experiencing their first episode of depression (Conwell et al., 2000; Lynch et al., 1999), and depressed older adults are much more likely than younger adults to act on suicidal thoughts and actually kill themselves (Kaplan, Adamek, and Rhoades, 1998). Accordingly, any evaluation of an older adult who has signs of depression should include an assessment of suicide risk. But identifying suicidal elders is not easy: Most who show "risk factors" for suicidal ideation or behavior (e.g., physical illness and functional disability, severe depressive symptoms, being widowed, divorced, or socially isolated) are not suicidal (Callahan et al., 1996).

The suicide of an older person often follows missed opportunities for prevention or early intervention (Kaplan, Adamek, and Calderon, 1999; Uncapher and Arean, 2000); indeed, about three-quarters of those who do commit suicide visit their primary care doctor within one month prior to the suicide (Conwell, 1994). Samuel's case shows that, even when depression is recognized as his was, inadequate coordination among too many systems of care can allow a bad situation to escalate into a worse one.

Samuel Schmitt: Introduction

Eighty-six-year-old Samuel Schmitt had a long history of insulin-dependent diabetes, obesity, and coronary artery disease. Ida, his wife of fifty-five years, had memory problems due to vascular dementia and her everyday functioning had changed dramatically over the past year. She stopped cooking, no longer called to talk to the grandchildren, and lost her usual humor and enthusiasm. Samuel's attempts to cook for them failed, so Ida's primary care nurse arranged "meals-on-wheels" delivery five days a week. Samuel tried to manage both his and Ida's multiple medications, but administering a combination of eleven medications across four different times of the day was no easy task.

When Ida's doctor recommended that she live someplace where she could get more care than Samuel was able to provide, their two sons who lived in distant states helped them to sell their home and move to St. Joseph's, an independent-living facility for seniors in the next town. The facility provided meals and, for an extra fee, a nurse to administer medications to Ida.

The move seemed to make Ida worse. Her repeated questions and clinging behavior tried Samuel's patience. Already feeling like a failure as a caregiver, he hated living in their single room, and missed his garage and his tools. He also missed making his own decisions; other people told him what to eat, when to eat, and even with whom to sit in the dining room. He felt he had lost everything: his wife, his house, his freedom.

Questioning at the time of his next scheduled physical exam revealed that Samuel was not managing his insulin consistently; he said he tried but didn't really care. His doctor told him he was depressed and prescribed sertraline (Zoloft). Samuel, reluctant to take more medication, only sometimes remembered it.

Some weeks later, Samuel woke up in the hospital. He had passed out due to unstable blood sugar levels. When he was discharged back to St. Joseph's, now with nursing assistance to monitor his medications and blood sugar, neither Samuel nor the staff realized that the hospital had inadvertently discontinued the Zoloft prescription.

Over the next few weeks, Samuel was feeling increasingly hopeless and helpless. He was bored, he knew he couldn't help his wife, and he couldn't think of a good reason to continue living this way; on a phone call with his son one day, he said the family would be better off without him. The son promptly called St. Joseph's. The charge nurse evaluated his suicidal intent and he was transferred for evaluation to the geropsychiatric unit at the local psychiatric hospital.

Issues for Consideration

Among the issues contributing to the complexity of the case are: multiple risks for suicidal depression, the importance of comprehensive assessment in geriatric care, and the potentially adverse depression outcomes associated with poor continuity of care. And among the issues contributing to Samuel's depression itself are: grief over his wife's illness and decline, loss of independence in his own home, decreased availability of previously enjoyed activities, multiple chronic illnesses complicated by poor adherence to his health care plan, and possible mild cognitive impairment affecting self-care. All of these factors will need to be addressed with continued evaluation.

Samuel's case shows how it is easy to miss opportunities for thorough assessment, which, when seized in a timely fashion, can lead to earlier interventions and prevention of acute psychiatric care. Such missed opportunities arose during the planning first of home care services and then of nursing help at the assisted living facility. In both settings, the focus was on Ida's needs; with no reference to the potential of depression and/or cognitive change to interfere, Samuel was incorrectly presumed to be able to monitor at least his own medications. It is important to remember that when the more obviously impaired member of an older couple becomes the "identified patient," the less obviously impaired spouse may not actually be a capable caregiver; indeed, s/he may be in need of services him/herself.

In the primary care setting, where Samuel's depression was properly if belatedly recognized, in-depth evaluation of contributing factors rarely occurs. Although his physician did initiate treatment by prescribing an antidepressant medication, essential questions remained unasked: Why was Samuel missing insulin doses? Because he forgot? Because he didn't realize how important it was to take regularly? Or, because he in fact did not care if his health deteriorated? Was

Samuel having problems with memory or other cognitive functions? How was he coping with the multiple losses he was enduring? Could he benefit from additional social services or psychotherapeutic support? Did he have thoughts about suicide at that time? (See Box 7.1 at the end of the chapter for a sample script on asking questions about a patient's suicidality.)

Poor continuity across treatment settings is a common risk in geriatric care. It did create problems in Samuel's case, and would need to be addressed in future treatment planning. Within several months' time, Samuel received outpatient and inpatient medical care, as well as home and residential care services. When Samuel's doctor prescribed antidepressant medication, there was no plan to assure that he would or could comply with this treatment when he got home, and this oversight led to its falling through the cracks completely when he was discharged from the hospital. Effective interventions initiated in one situation are useless without supports for follow-through and, because our care system is not designed to facilitate seamless care across settings, frail older adults without close supervision by capable family or friends are at higher risk for adverse outcomes.

Assessment

At the hospital admission unit, Samuel met with a psychologist for about an hour. He spoke softly and slowly, mostly stared at the floor, and became tearful on several occasions. With questioning he admitted to her that he was feeling helpless, hopeless, and worthless, and was enjoying little about living. He said that his thoughts of suicide were more and more frequent and intense so that now he could think of almost nothing else. He had planned to end his life that night after his wife went to bed, by overdosing on all of his medications. He could not think of a reason to live, and repeated that ending his life would be "best for everyone." His only concern about this plan was disgrace to his sons. He denied any prior suicidal thoughts or attempts in his life, nor could he recall prior experiences of depression.

The psychologist briefly evaluated his cognitive status with a Mini-Mental State Exam screen, and found that his concentration and verbal recall appeared impaired (MMSE = 23/30). Once Samuel's depression was under control, further cognitive assessment would be necessary to rule out early dementia since it was difficult to determine whether the screening deficits reflected only the severe depression or signified a more long-standing memory problem.

The psychologist explained to Samuel that he appeared to be severely depressed and that his level of hopelessness raised concerns about his safety; she said she believed he needed to stay in the psychiatric hospital for a short time, but that patients like him typically transferred into the partial-hospitalization program after a brief inpatient stay. Though Samuel wasn't happy about being in another hospital, he admitted some relief at having someone recognize his despair and agreed to the admission.

Conceptualization

Samuel's case is one where interacting biological, psychological, and social risk factors all played a part in his increasingly severe depression—and his eventual feeling that suicide was the only solution to his predicament.

His diabetes and coronary artery disease needed consistent care to optimize his physical strength, energy, and cognition. So did the antidepressant medication: His discharge plan would need to include monitoring of his response to it and adjustments made as necessary.

Samuel was struggling with grief from the layered losses of his home, his independence, his wife as he knew her, and his sense of usefulness and worth. He needs help to regain some of the key aspects of his identity. Further cognitive evaluation to help sort out his strengths and weaknesses would allow realistic planning for his care and activities.

Samuel felt isolated and useless at St. Joseph's and needed extra support to identify meaningful activities or relationships. While his inpatient and partial-hospital mental health treatments could provide such support initially, discharge plans had to consider forums for him to maintain feelings of self-worth and enjoyment despite his changing abilities and roles. A plan reflecting clear communication and continuity of care among settings was also crucial.

Treatment

Samuel was voluntarily admitted to the geropsychiatric unit for five days. The psychiatrist restarted him on Zoloft. The nurses supervised Samuel's diabetes care (administering insulin and checking sugars). The social worker spoke with Samuel's sons and the staff at St. Joseph's to identify resources/supports that would be important upon his return there. Samuel attended group classes on the unit's day program (exercise, group therapy, methods of self-change, leisure management, goal setting, coping with change, and devotions).

At first his participation was minimal, but the group leaders helped him to identify the stressors contributing to his depression. At the end of the fifth day, he was discharged from the inpatient unit back to St. Joseph's to return the next morning for classes in the partial-hospitalization program, which met weekdays from 9 A.M. to 3 P.M. St. Joseph's would continue to provide nursing supervision for his medications. Meanwhile, Samuel also agreed to a referral for neuropsychological testing.

Samuel attended the same day program classes he had while an inpatient, and became an increasingly active group participant. He appreciated learning that he was not alone, meeting other older adults dealing with difficult transitions and losses, and making them laugh with the kind of humor Ida was no longer able to appreciate. After the first week of classes, he felt ready to face the weekend at St. Joseph's. He planned to attend Sunday church service, as well as a meeting of residents organizing to volunteer in the local high school industrial arts class. After two weeks, Samuel reduced his partial hospital treatment from five to three days per week and continued there for another month. Over time in the program, he was able to talk some about his years of work, military, family, religious, and community experience, which—with interest and validation from others—helped to remind him that his life was more than the sum of his current illnesses. He also felt supported by others who had experienced grief when a spouse got sick or died.

Neuropsychological testing found that he had verbal retrieval and executive functioning deficits consistent with a mild vascular dementia. He needed cues to help his memory and structure to help him follow through with activities. The partial-hospital program worked with Samuel and the staff of St. Joseph's to design a weekly schedule that he could post in his room and be encouraged to follow. After "graduating" from the day program, Samuel continued to see a social worker every two–three weeks for monitoring and support and to see his psychiatrist quarterly. Samuel never embraced the changes in his life, but he was able to make the best of his situation by enjoying some of his activities and relationships with other residents and staff and deriving spiritual comfort from renewed participation with his church. He also felt strongly about being there for Ida (despite her changes, she still took comfort in his presence) and showing courage to his sons and grandchildren.

Comment

Samuel had a good initial response to the recognition of his despair and the safety and structure provided by the acute hospitalization. His relatively quick response to the group partial-hospital program illustrates how important interpersonal support, validation, and structure can be for an older person—particularly for one who feels isolated and overwhelmed by changes in familiar roles, relationships, and/or living situations. Meeting with other elders can serve to normalize feelings of grief and allow expression and appreciation of the stable aspects of oneself. Further, supporting many elders' connection to religious or spiritual coping can be important (Koenig, George, and Siegler, 1988; Ramsey and Blieszner, 2000).

Samuel's experience was not typical in that his county had a psychiatric hospital with an excellent continuum of geriatric mental health services. Ordinarily, acute psychiatric hospitalization—which certainly should serve as a "wake-up call" for improved care coordination—does not guarantee that a comprehensive discharge plan appropriate to the elder's multiple needs will be put into place. Geriatric partial-hospitalization programs provide an important transition for elders recovering from acute psychiatric illness and can also be used to help to prevent psychiatric inpatient hospitalization.

It is important to note that outcomes with suicidal older adults are frequently more tragic. Samuel had many of the risk factors for suicide, being a white man over the age of 80 with health-related disability, recent loss, severe depression, and feelings of hopelessness. Had he had access to a gun and a more impulsive style, or had he lacked the support of his alert son, he may have committed suicide. Asking elders about access to firearms is critical, as they are the most common suicide method among both older men and older women in the United States (Kaplan, Adamek, and Rhoades, 1998).

One final note about suicidality in late life: Is late-life suicide ever rational and, if so, under what circumstances? This is a difficult question. Many older adults wish to have some control over the nature of their death, fearing severe disability, pain, mental incapacity, or lack of dignity at the end of life. Capable adults have the right to refuse unwanted life-sustaining medical treatments and many of us might choose to limit aggressive medical interventions in the face of terminal illness (Karel, 2000). Most terminally ill patients, however, do *not* express suicidal thoughts or request active assistance to die; those who do desire a hastened death are very likely to suffer from depression (Breitbart et al., 2000).

Although cases exist in which suicidal wishes reflect a rational decision to end suffering rather than depression or other reversible despair, it is critical that suicidal thoughts in disabled older adults not be considered "reasonable" as a matter of course. Most frail elders do not express a desire to hasten their death and, when such sentiments are expressed, it usually reflects an unmet need (e.g., pain control, social support, spiritual suffering). Evaluation by a mental health professional can be very helpful in these circumstances (Block and Billings, 1995), and every effort should be made to address the patient's physical, psychological, and spiritual comfort (Tobin, 1998).

BOX 7.1 Asking the Depressed Older Adult About Suicidality

Do not be afraid to ask older clients about thoughts of suicide. They accept such inquiries when made with a matter-of-fact attitude and respectful concern for the individual. Important elements to include are: past and present suicidal thoughts, plans, and attempts; access to weapons; reasons for living and reasons for not acting on suicidal thoughts. Be direct, ask questions in different ways, and avoid the temptation to ask questions in the negative (e.g., "You're not thinking of killing yourself, are you?"). Here is a script that Samuel's physician might have used on recognizing Samuel's depression, which might have allowed for earlier intervention.

MD: Sam, I can see it has been a very difficult few months for you with Ida's illness and the move and all. You've said that sometimes you just don't care anymore. Have you ever felt so bad the past few weeks that you thought you'd prefer to die?

Sam: Whenever God wants me, I'm ready to go.

MD: Have you thought you would want to hasten your death, to take your own life?

Sam: I don't know.

MD: Sometimes people feel so hopeless that suicide feels like the only option. Have you ever had that feeling, in the past or recently?

Sam: Well, I certainly never felt that before, I could always handle everything. Lately, it just doesn't seem worth it. What good am I, a sick old man?

MD: What thoughts have you had about taking your life?

Sam: Well, I figure all those medications could put me to sleep forever.

MD: You thought about taking all of your medications?

Sam: Well, I thought of it, but don't think I could do it.

MD: Have you ever taken too many of your medicines?

Sam: No, at least not on purpose. I know I forget sometimes if I took my dose.

MD: Yes, let's talk about your memory concerns in a few minutes. Let me ask you, what would keep you from overdosing on all your medicines?

Sam: I don't want my sons to remember me that way.

MD: Do you have any other means of hurting yourself at the facility, like a gun or other weapon?

Sam: No, I got rid of my gun years ago. They wouldn't let me keep something like that there anyway. I don't even have my tools anymore.

MD: Sam, can you think of any reason that you would want to continue to live? Is there anything that makes life worth living?

(continues)

BOX 7.1 (continued)

Sam: Well, Ida was always the main reason, but now there's nothing I can do to help her. I always like seeing my sons and their families, but they both live so far, it's hard waiting for those visits once or twice a year, but I guess that has kept me going. I just wish I could concentrate on reading, at least I should be able to do that.

MD: As we discussed earlier, I believe you are suffering from depression, which is a serious illness we can help you with. Your depression could be affecting your concentration for reading, as well as making you feel like life offers no pleasure anymore. Sometimes when people are very depressed, they feel like giving up; that is not uncommon. I am concerned about you and would like to suggest that we arrange regular contact with a counselor who might be able to help you find things to do at St. Joseph's, as well as monitor how you are doing with the antidepressant medicine I am suggesting for you. Would you be willing to try that?

Sam: If that's what you think, doc, sure.

MD: It also might help to see if a nurse can help you with your medicines at St. Joseph's, given your concerns about your memory and just to be on the safe side. Would it be OK if I called the director there and let her know about our conversation here today?

Sam: Well I don't want her to think I'm crazy.

MD: I don't think you're crazy, nor will she. I just want to do what we can to keep you healthy and safe while we work to help you with the depression you've been having. The nurse director there is very familiar with wanting to help people with depression. Believe me, you're not alone with this problem. Is it OK if I talk with her?

Sam: Sure, I guess you want to help.

MD: I'll see you again in a month and we can see how you're doing then. When your depression clears up a bit, which often takes several months, I'd like to talk to you some more about your memory and maybe we can get that checked out too.

CHAPTER EIGHT

Chronic Illness, Anxiety, and Depression: Arnie Price

Older adults with chronic illness often face changes in their strength, stamina, sensory acuity, or surefootedness, which can make it difficult and sometimes frightening to carry out usual daily activities. Realistic fears—or simply realistic appraisal of one's abilities—lead many older adults to limit their activities. In the extreme, fears are exaggerated and an older person can become excessively disabled by anxiety and avoidance of positive activity. Symptoms of anxiety, depression, and chronic medical illness often overlap (e.g., concentration troubles, sleep disturbance, ruminative worry, restlessness, somatic discomfort, and restriction of activity) and can be difficult to distinguish in older patients. In fact, depressed elders often have prominent anxiety symptoms or disorders, while anxious elders often develop depressive symptoms (Beck and Stanley, 1997; Flint, 1994; Lenze et al., 2000; Shapiro, Roberts, and Beck, 1999). Appropriate treatment depends on thorough assessment of the relative prominence of depression, anxiety, and other symptoms in the older adult. In Arnie's case, his pulmonary illness was frightening and limiting and led to both anxiety and depression.

Arnie Price: Introduction

> Arnie was a 68-year-old, divorced, previously active and energetic man who was diagnosed with chronic obstructive pulmonary disease (COPD) at the age of 62. He finally quit smoking when the illness was diagnosed. Over the past three years, his stamina had become so poor that he was increasingly reluctant to do much of anything. He was frightened when he

could not catch his breath, and tired easily with short walks or household chores; occasionally he panicked when he was out shopping and pushing himself to maintain his pace. In the past year, he quit his part-time driving delivery job, and rarely went out to the bowling alley or his favorite coffee shop. He also was cutting down his visits to his daughter Liz and her family.

At his last medical appointment, he told his doctor that he was feeling nervous, tired, and not himself. She asked if he was making an effort to exercise, and he explained he was afraid to exert himself. She advised him to walk slowly a short distance each day, and also gave him a prescription for lorazepam (Ativan). The medicine did help calm his nerves a bit, but he still didn't feel like getting out or making the effort to walk. Liz was increasingly concerned about his inactivity and isolation, and asked a therapist she knew for some advice. The therapist recommended a local psychologist, and Liz talked to her dad about going in for an evaluation.

Issues for Consideration

Accurate diagnosis of psychiatric illness can be difficult in an older person suffering from disabling medical illness and symptoms of anxiety and depression. With this limited information about Arnie, we can begin to wonder: Is he suffering from an anxiety disorder, a depressive disorder, neither, or both? Does he have panic disorder? Agoraphobia? Generalized anxiety? Major depression? An adjustment disorder? Or, simply, a normal reaction to physical changes? In many cases, the older adult's combination of symptoms will not fit neatly into a DSM-IV diagnostic category. However, continued assessment will help to sort out some of these questions.

When an older person with chronic medical illness suffers psychiatric symptoms, the first question always needs to be whether the illness is being optimally treated and/or whether any of the treatments may contribute to behavioral symptoms. Further, we need to know how the individual is adhering to the prescribed treatments. Collaboration with medical care providers is important in this context.

Individuals differ in their strategies for coping with illness and disability. For example, those whose self-esteem is directly tied to their physical capacity may have more trouble adapting to bodily changes than those whose self-esteem is based largely in their capacity for interpersonal relations. In Arnie's case, what about his personality or coping style may affect his adaptation to a difficult and disabling illness?

Assessment

Arnie had no prior psychiatric problems or experience with mental health treatment. He was embarrassed to call the "shrink" recommended by his daughter, and nervous about physically getting to the office at the medical center in town. But, he realized he needed some kind of help. He told Liz he'd handle it on his own, knowing she was busy with work and the kids. Two weeks after he made the call, he went to his appointment. The psychologist introduced herself, described what would happen in the meeting, and asked Arnie what brought him in.

Arnie said his daughter thought he should come in, that he had been feeling awful physically, had trouble breathing, couldn't walk, and was not able to leave the house except for occasional errands. He was starting to feel like a burden to his daughter. He had given up most of his activities, and felt bored, angry, and useless. He couldn't believe what had become of his life.

During the course of the evaluation, the psychologist asked Arnie about his medical and social history, and current patterns of anxiety and depression symptoms. He signed a release allowing her to contact his primary care and pulmonary physicians, who treated him for COPD, hypertension, and benign prostate hypertrophy. He took several medications daily: prednisone, inhalers, a hypertension medication, and Ativan. When the psychologist later called the pulmonary doctor, he confirmed that recent pulmonary function tests were as good as could be expected and that Arnie was doing well on the prednisone; he had not noticed Arnie to have any adverse behavioral reactions common with that medication. The pulmonologist expressed concern that Arnie was not attempting any exercise and felt that his physical limitations were greater than expected given his pulmonary status.

In the interview, Arnie disclosed symptoms of both anxiety and depression, including: almost constant worry about his health and breathing, concern with multiple physical symptoms, approximately three or four anxiety attacks per month (reduced from several per week since he limited his activity), decreased energy, decreased concentration for reading and television, loss of interest in usual activities, decreased motivation, irritability/impatience, feeling useless, feeling worthless, and restless sleep. He was eating fine, maintained a sense of humor, had some hope that things could improve, and had no thoughts about suicide. He had no prior treatment for anxiety or depression. Although he admitted to feeling very sad and stressed both when his marriage was ending and, more recently, when his ex-wife died, he said he was always able to keep busy and rely on work, bowling, and friends for distraction.

The psychologist also learned that Arnie had been an energetic, somewhat rushed and pressured guy who liked to drive fast, walk fast, and talk fast. He had always been busy with something. This slowing down and lack of activity did not feel comfortable to him at all. With further questioning, Arnie shared that he had no history of trauma and no family history of psychiatric problems. A high school graduate, he had worked many hours in his printing business, and described good relationships with his adult daughter and son.

Arnie told the psychologist that talking to her wasn't as bad as he had expected, and agreed to return the following week. As requested, he completed the Geriatric Depression Scale and Beck Anxiety Inventory at home in the interim. During their second meeting, review of these scales showed moderate symptoms of both depression and anxiety (GDS = 13/30; BAI=21/63).

After discussing the scale scores with him, the psychologist introduced Arnie to the concept of the relationship between mood, thoughts, and behaviors. So that they could both learn more about his experiences over time, she asked him to monitor his mood each day on a form they created together (both depression, where 1 = very depressed/sad and 10 = very happy, and anxiety, where 1 = very nervous/worried and 10 = very relaxed) and describe why he thought he felt that way (Zeiss and Steffen, 1996). She also asked him to note any incidents of anxiety attacks and specific information about it on the form: when and where it happened and what he was thinking and doing before, during, and after the attack. Together, they practiced rating his mood and describing his most recent anxiety attack.

Arnie was relatively motivated and able to complete these assignments. He rated his anxiety levels consistently at a 6 or a 7 on days he stayed home, and worse on the two days he had gone out—once to the grocery store and once to his daughter's (2 or 3). He indicated that he felt more anxious on those days because he had to walk a bit. He reported one anxiety "attack," in which he felt very frightened, immobilized, and embarrassed, when he was returning from his car to his apartment, rushing to get to the toilet. He said he was thinking he might wet himself and that he'd be embarrassed if anyone saw him, and that he felt relieved once he made it into his apartment and to the toilet. He rated depression consistently at a 6, except for a 3 on the day of the anxiety attack.

The psychologist's impression was that Arnie was suffering primarily from anxiety secondary to COPD, with occasional breathing-related anxiety/panic attacks and avoidance of activity that might cause him to panic. He did not appear to have a major depressive disorder, but was suffering mild depression secondary to his anxiety and functional limitations. The psychologist's impression was also that Arnie had many resources to help him feel better: motivation, intelligence, a sense of humor, support from his children, and previous involvement in social and other activities.

Conceptualization

Arnie, although initially reluctant to seek mental health treatment, was motivated to participate in a behavioral assessment of his anxiety symptoms. He did not want to be a burden on others; this collaborative assessment–and treatment–fit well with his "take-charge" style. The psychologist was careful to check with Arnie's medical care providers to ensure that additional medical interventions were not currently necessary. Arnie's premorbid high-energy, high-pressure personality style likely made coping with this debilitating illness all the more difficult for him. The initial treatment plan included helping Arnie to understand the connection between his symptoms and activity level; to accept and learn strategies to cope with activity limitations secondary to COPD; to identify and increase participation in activities he could continue to do (and, thus, his sense of control and purpose); and to review his use of anxiety-reducing medication.

Treatment

Arnie agreed to return weekly for approximately ten meetings for cognitive-behavioral psychotherapy with the psychologist, as well as to consultation with a psychiatrist.

The psychotherapy treatment focused initially on teaching Arnie about the relationship between anxiety, his physical symptoms, and his behaviors. He continued to keep his anxiety log, maintaining it on the old computer his daughter had given him. He realized that he was afraid of physical symptoms and, as he avoided activity, he became physically weaker, more susceptible to physical stress, and bored and depressed.

Arnie needed help learning to slow down. When he did try to walk, get out, or do chores, he felt a pressure to move quickly and inevitably became very anxious. He was able to practice behavioral techniques to pace himself. For example, when walking, he worked to accept that he had to move slowly and took to repeating mantras to himself, such as "go slow, it's OK to go slow." He made efforts to take slow breaths with the first signs of escalating anxiety. He also practiced stopping and resting frequently, and worked to tell himself that this was a sign of intelligent adaptation rather than weakness. He struggled with feeling embarrassed about his disability, but tried using a combination of humor and honesty when he felt he needed to explain himself to someone ("I'm just a man with bad lungs who needs to stop to catch his breath, I'll get there eventually").

Having dropped most of his usual activities, Arnie also needed help to realistically appraise what activities he could do and enjoy on his own, what activities he could no longer do, and what activities he could do with help. While practicing walking more slowly, he realized he could still visit his daughter's family for dinner once a week and meet the guys at the coffee shop. Although it was difficult, he tried to walk a short distance in the mall most days, and used the benches there when he needed to rest. He was also enjoying the computer, and decided to take a computer class at the library: He felt fine when sitting and it didn't tire him to move his fingers! Consequently, as he increased these activities, his depressive symptoms started to decrease.

At the same time, Arnie decided that he could not realistically return to his bowling league and did not feel up to resuming his part-time job. Finally, he knew he needed to do something about his apartment. He was typically rather clean, but easily tired now when vacuuming, dusting, organizing, or washing, and had let his place deteriorate. Admitting he needed help, the place got cleaned with his daughter's assistance and a few hours of paid help. With the psychologist's encouragement, he was trying to learn that asking for help when he needed it was one way of taking control of the situation, rather than an admission of helplessness. This was not easy, but he was trying.

In addition to the psychotherapy, Arnie saw a psychiatrist. They decided to taper him off his regular Ativan prescription, but that he could take it as needed if feeling very anxious. The psychiatrist also explained other, safer medication options (such as SSRIs or buspirone), but Arnie was encouraged about the progress he had made in psychotherapy and decided not to start a new medication.

Over several months, Arnie reported decreased symptoms of anxiety (BAI = 12) and depression (GDS = 7), and only one incident of a panic attack. Although he remained frustrated and discouraged by his physical limitations at times, he no longer reported feeling helpless, hopeless, or worthless. After three months of weekly psychotherapy meetings and follow-up psychiatric consultation, Arnie decided to schedule several bimonthly psychotherapy appointments to reinforce his efforts and gains and to follow up with the psychiatrist in six months. The psychologist reassured him that, if he faced difficulties down the road, he should not hesitate to call.

Comment

Arnie was a very motivated client, despite his initial reluctance to engage in mental health treatment. His usual take-charge style and solid foundation of interests and relationships helped him to cope with his anxiety and depression. Many older individuals who experience anxiety and/or depression in the context of disability are effective collaborators in skills-based cognitive-behavioral interventions. Previous strengths and resources can be applied to new problems.

Some older clients, especially those with mild cognitive deficits affecting initiation or concentration, may have difficulty with cognitive-behavioral monitoring and skill-building. Other individuals may have emotional difficulty taking such an active role in helping themselves to get better, such as those with passive personality styles, those who are seeking attention or caring through the sick role, or those whose anxiety or depression is severe. In such cases, addressing these barriers more directly is important. In addition, in cases where individuals have difficulty experimenting with new behaviors, family members or other caregivers can be included in the treatment to help cue or reinforce adaptive behaviors.

In working with chronically ill elders, selected interventions also depend in part on the severity and progression of the individual's illness. Arnie had a progressive illness that was likely to be increasingly disabling over the years. However, at the time of this treatment, his medical condition was generally stable and his anxiety and depression were causing excess disability. If he had been a person who expressed specific fears for the future, or if he was no longer able to live independently, the therapy may have focused more on issues of grief and facing end-of-life concerns.

CHAPTER NINE

Chronic Pain and Depression: Lillian Green

Many medical problems common in late life can cause chronic pain (e.g., osteoarthritis, peripheral vascular disease, diabetes) (Ferrell and Ferrell, 1996). Chronic pain and depression are related, with depression both resulting from and contributing to the experience of pain (Gloth, 2000; Ostbye et al., 2000) and exacerbated by the consequences of interrupted sleep and inhibited activity (Muldovsky and Scarisbrick, 1976; Scudds and Robertson, 1998). Limitations in activity can result from the actual physical disability, pain, fear, reduced self-efficacy, or feelings of embarrassment or shame. In Lillian's case, osteoarthritis, urinary incontinence, hypothyroidism, and complications of diabetes combined to affect negatively her sleep, activity level, and social contacts and, ultimately, led to major depression. She was helped by careful medical and pain management, physical therapy, and problem-solving therapy in the primary care setting.

Lillian Green: Introduction

Lillian was a 70-year-old retired schoolteacher who had been living alone since her husband's death from lung cancer six years earlier. Since that time, she kept fairly active visiting her friends and swimming in the local pool twice per week. She had frequent phone contact with her daughter, son, and their families, and managed to see them every few months although they lived in distant states.

Lillian was being treated for a number of chronic medical conditions, including hypothyroidism, hypertension, non-insulin-dependent diabetes, and osteoarthritis in both hips. Over the past year, she also developed mild urinary incontinence and had several episodes where she was not able to control her bladder when in public places such as the grocery store or the library. Concerned and embarrassed, but reluctant to mention the problem to her primary care provider or her children, Lillian was staying home more, avoiding trips to see friends, to use the pool, or even to run errands.

At her next primary care visit, the physician—who had treated Lillian for the past ten years—noticed that she seemed less talkative than usual. Her blood sugar was elevated and Lillian seemed frustrated about her difficulty keeping the sugar levels under control despite starting a new oral diabetic medicine several months ago. She stated that maybe it wasn't worth it for them to worry so much about the blood sugar, because nothing seemed to work and she was just getting old anyway. She complained that worsening right hip pain was keeping her from sleeping through the night. She also mentioned that she was having problems controlling her bladder. The physician, who had spent the past 15 minutes addressing her other chronic medical problems, was concerned about the urinary incontinence and discussed with Lillian a number of diagnostic tests that could help evaluate the cause of this problem.

He also briefly entertained the thought that Lillian might be depressed, although he had not ever known her to be so. When he asked her directly, she expressed frustration instead about her multiple medical problems. Understanding her frustration at feeling so unable to control them, he focused on recommendations for managing the diabetes—increasing the oral hypoglycemic medication—and controlling the pain—starting a new nonsteroidal pain medication. He also prescribed a low dose of Trazodone to help her with sleep at night and referred her to a urologist to evaluate the urinary incontinence. He asked her to return in one month for a follow-up.

Issues for Consideration

Lillian's primary care visit illustrates the real challenge for diagnosing depression in the face of multiple medical problems, medications, and chronic pain. In this contact, the physician was wondering whether Lillian was depressed, and even asked her about it, but she minimized that concern and emphasized the difficulty she was having with her multiple physical problems. With so many issues to address in this one meeting, it is easy to understand how a more extensive depression evaluation did not occur. What might have helped the doctor and/or Lillian to pursue concerns about depression in this meeting?

Fortunately, the primary doctor asked to see her again quite soon so he would have another opportunity to see how she was doing.

Assessment

When Lillian returned to her doctor four weeks later, her right hip pain was somewhat improved but was still bothering her at night and limiting her ability to go out and get exercise. Plus, she said her feet were hurting her more lately, making it even more uncomfortable to walk. Her blood sugar was improved on the higher dose of medication. She had not followed up on the referral to the urologist because she said she did not have the time or energy to do so. She also admitted that she was afraid the urologist might suggest surgery, which she felt she could not tolerate at her age; she recalled a difficult surgery with some complications following her second pregnancy.

Lillian had lost eight pounds since her last visit; she complained of poor appetite and energy, and expressed continued frustration about her persistent pain and urinary incontinence. The physician ordered several blood tests to rule out possible worsening hypothyroidism, anemia or an electrolyte imbalance (both of which could be caused by medications she was taking), and long-term blood glucose control. He also administered the 15-item version of the Geriatric Depression

Scale (GDS), on which she scored in the moderately depressed range (9/15 points). She endorsed depressed mood, difficulty pursuing or enjoying activities that used to give her pleasure, feelings of worthlessness and helplessness, low energy, and not feeling in good spirits. She denied problems with her memory or, with further questioning, any suicidal ideation. The doctor suggested that she might be suffering from a major depressive episode and discussed possible treatments, including antidepressant medication or a course of psychotherapy. As Lillian was reluctant to start yet another medication, the physician encouraged her to see a psychiatric social worker who was affiliated with his practice.

The social worker called Lillian the next day to schedule an appointment for the following week. During that meeting, the social worker asked her for more information about her history, current stressors, and social supports. Lillian described her demoralization about feeling so limited by her pain, her fear of wetting herself, and her overall poor energy. She had always been an active, independent, motivated, and intellectually curious woman, had enjoyed her career as a primary school teacher, and, after retiring at the age of 60, had volunteered giving swimming lessons to disabled children. She stopped that when her husband got sick. His cancer was diagnosed at a relatively late stage and he died within a year.

She coped reasonably well after his death, with support from extended family and friends, and had adjusted to life on her own. Her closest supports were her sister who lived nearby, several girlfriends, and her children. However, with all her physical problems over the past year, Lillian was spending less time with these people and now feeling lonely. Lillian could recall one prior experience of depression, after a difficult childbirth and subsequent surgery and complications. She received no treatment for depression at the time but recalled that she had slowly felt better over the period of a year.

Conceptualization

Clearly, multiple medical issues are contributing to Lillian's depression. Her hip pain is contributing to poor sleep and reduced activity, both of which make her feel more tired, useless, and depressed. With little activity to distract her, she sits at home and thinks more about her worsening pain. In addition to the arthritic hip pain, she is likely experiencing lower extremity pain from diabetic neuropathy, which has not yet been addressed. Lillian is caught in a common vicious cycle of pain–poor sleep–depression–increasing physical limitations. For Lillian, this cycle is made even worse by the onset of urinary incontinence, causing her to avoid outside activity and thus become increasingly homebound. Other medical problems, such as hypothyroidism or anemia, as addressed by the physician, could also contribute to depressive symptoms.

Lillian, used to being an active, capable, and sociable woman, has become essentially disabled and, as she stays home more, she is also withdrawing from her usual social supports. She now sees her sister and friends less often and, although they call and drop by at times, she feels less up to talking with them. In keeping with a common depressive cycle, Lillian's apparent disinterest may be offputting to her friends who eventually call on her less often.

Her treatment will have to address this range of medical and social issues.

Treatment

Lillian had six meetings with the psychiatric social worker and completed a course of problem-solving treatment in primary care (PST-PC) (Hegel, Barrett, and Oxman, 2000). They worked together to identify, and find ways to overcome, the primary contributors to Lillian's depression and excess disability (i.e., becoming more socially isolated, stopping most of her activities, focusing more on her pain). The social worker encouraged Lillian to obtain the urological evaluation and helped her to see that fear of surgery was preventing her from collecting information that might suggest other solutions for her incontinence. The urologist referred Lillian for physical therapy to learn exercises to help control her relatively mild urinary incontinence. With the help of the physical therapist and her social worker, she was also referred to and joined a support group for women with urinary incontinence. In this setting, Lillian learned to be less embarrassed to talk about the problem and to go out despite it, with the help of both her exercises and an absorbent pad.

The social worker also encouraged Lillian to call her friends and let them know she had been having a hard time, but wanted to make an effort to get out. Lillian was not comfortable with the idea of "complaining," but realized her friends did care about her and she'd want her friends to come to her if they needed extra support or encouragement. With the social worker, Lillian listed the activities she most missed and wanted to try to return to: weekly trips to the library, card games with her friends, and swimming at the pool. She slowly made an effort to reengage with these activities, particularly with her physician's ongoing help to cope with the pain. He too sent Lillian to a physical therapist, and she was delighted to learn that pool-based exercises could be palliative for her osteoarthritis. He switched her pain medications to a regular, rather than as-needed, dosing schedule, and he consulted with a psychiatrist who recommended a low dose of venlafaxine (Effexor) to help with residual depressive symptoms plus the pain from diabetic neuropathy.

Over the next two months, Lillian started to feel more like her old self again. She knew her arthritis slowed her down, but she was nonetheless spending more time out of the house, pushing herself to continue activities that she could, and seeing her family and friends. She was sleeping better at night and not feeling as exhausted during the day. Her appetite came back and she was again able to enjoy lunch out with friends several times a week. She continued quarterly visits with her primary care doctor.

Comment

Lillian's case speaks to the difficulty of diagnosing depression in the context of multiple medical problems, as well as to the excess disability caused by depression and the significant improvement in functioning that its treatment can bring about. Lillian was fortunate to have a primary care physician who knew her over time, who was attentive to the possibility of depression, and who encouraged her to follow up with psychotherapy as well as specialty medical evaluation (urology) and physical therapy. He was also attentive to her concerns about pain, which should always be assessed and taken seriously (Tait, 1999).

The mental health referral was facilitated by having a psychiatric social worker in the primary care practice. She was easily able to collaborate with the primary care physician and could provide quick and accessible follow-up with the patient (see models of care described in Appendix C).

Although late-life medical problems and their associated disabilities and indignities can be difficult to accept, most older adults find ways to adapt their activities and their expectations so that they can continue to enjoy what they are still able to do. Depression interferes with this capacity to adapt; appropriate treatment can restore it and improve the quality of life.

CHAPTER TEN

Anxiety, Depression, and Benzodiazepine Dependence: Geneva Sampson

When older adults indicate to their doctors that they are having trouble with their nerves, worries, or sleep, they are often prescribed sedative or anxiolytic (anxiety-reducing) medications. Because symptoms of depression and anxiety commonly co-occur in older patients (Beck and Stanley, 1997; Flint, 1994; Shapiro, Roberts, and Beck, 1999), anxiety symptoms can appear prominent and medications are often prescribed to address the anxiety. However, most anxiolytic medications do not treat underlying depression and carry the risk of increased tolerance, increased use, and physical or cognitive side effects that put elders at increased risk for injury (Center for Substance Abuse Treatment, 1998). Geneva's experience illustrates how an anxious older woman was treated with a benzodiazepine through her local emergency room, while her underlying depression and psychosocial stresses were not addressed. Her dependence on the medication ultimately led to injury, medical/surgical hospitalization, and, finally, appropriate treatment for her anxiety, depression, and psychosocial concerns.

Geneva Sampson: Introduction

> Geneva was a 79-year-old African-American woman who, though having lived independently in her apartment for many years, was becoming less comfortable living there on her own. She had developed several health problems—arthritis in her knees, congestive heart failure, and occasional dizziness—and

felt increasingly lonely, sad, and afraid. She had trouble getting in and out of the bathtub, and had almost fallen several times. She became fearful at nighttime, when she was sometimes bothered by waves of anxiety, chest pain, a racing heart, dizziness, diaphoresis (i.e., sweating), and shortness of breath. On these occasions, she went to the emergency room (ER), just a block away, and was reminded to take her Lasix (a diuretic to remove extra water from the body). Twice, the ER staff admitted her overnight to administer intravenous medicine to remove excess fluid from her body that was making it difficult for her to breathe. Though Geneva had a family doctor whom she saw every few months, she found it easiest to go to the local emergency room when she was scared.

During her third visit to the ER in four weeks, Geneva was diagnosed with an anxiety disorder and prescribed alprazolam (Xanax) 0.5 mg to take as she needed, up to four times a day. Initially, the medicine took the edge off her nerves but, over time, it was not working as well. On her next visit to the ER, she was told that she looked medically stable, to increase her dose of Xanax to 1 mg three times daily, and to follow up with her primary care provider. Again, she was relieved when the medicine helped her calm down.

During this time, Geneva ruminated about her situation: growing old, living alone, moving slower, being apart from her kids, and losing her sister and several friends during the past five years. As she and her siblings had cared for their aged parents in their homes, she was troubled that none of her three surviving children or ten grandchildren offered to do the same for her. She started thinking that maybe she was not worthy or loved, and didn't see much point in God letting her live if she was going to be alone and scared all the time. As her breathing troubles, dizziness, fear, and sadness continued, she took additional amounts of the Xanax without getting input from a medical provider.

One Saturday evening, she was feeling more anxious and took several pills. As she was getting into the tub for a bath, in preparation for church on Sunday, she fell and could not get up.

When her ride for church came to pick her up, they found her lying on the bathroom floor, where she had spent the night. An ambulance took her to the hospital and she received treatment for a broken hip.

Issues for Consideration

Geneva went so regularly to the ER that, in many ways, it had become her center for primary care. Her anxiety was eventually diagnosed there, but she developed increased tolerance to the Xanax that was prescribed and, as she used more of it to achieve the same calming effect, she was at increased risk for the injury that ultimately occurred. Questions we have include: In addition to being anxious, is she depressed? How dependent has she become on the Xanax? How are her physical health symptoms (e.g., congestive heart failure) exacerbating or contributing to her psychiatric symptoms? And, how are her psychiatric symptoms contributing to her physical health problems? What is her relationship like with her children, grandchildren, and other social supports? What has helped Geneva to cope during prior difficult times?

Assessment

During the first day of her hospitalization, Geneva frequently requested Xanax and maintained that the amount she received was inadequate; thus, she was referred for an evaluation by a consulting psychiatrist. She was agreeable to participate in the interview because she understood that the psychiatrist would give her the medication she needed to relax. The psychiatrist interviewed her at bedside, and found her to be an overweight, neatly groomed (she had made effort to put on lipstick even in the hospital), and proud but very distressed woman. She was tearful at times, and kept repeating her disbelief that her nerves had become so bad in her old age.

The psychiatrist asked her questions about her background. Geneva was the seventh of eight children, had a sixth grade education, and had worked cleaning houses. She married at age 17, and had four boys. Her husband died suddenly in his forties;

she and her sons managed with the support of her family. Now, six of her seven siblings had died and her youngest brother lived an hour away. Geneva had survived the death of her second son from cancer in his late twenties. Even so, she perceived her life as a good one: She had the support of friends and church, and had ten grandkids and seven great-grandchildren who were "good and hardworking."

Six years ago, her eldest son John was transferred to the East Coast with his company. Before John's move, he had visited her daily; her other two sons, one single and one divorced, lived within two-hour drives. Geneva saw John as her responsible son and, although he had married a woman whom the family disliked, he held the family together; it was at his house that they all gathered for holidays and birthdays. Geneva told the psychiatrist that, after John moved, it was her church and friends that kept her going, but that illness or death of several friends in the past five years meant grief and a smaller social network over time.

When asked about her grandchildren, Geneva brightened. She said they were the light of her life, and talked about how they were scattered all throughout the United States. She had two grandchildren in the area. However, her grandson (who had a wife and three small children) was busy with his job and family, and her granddaughter had many physical and financial problems, so their contact was limited.

Geneva attended church regularly and sang in the church choir, which she enjoyed. But with her weight gain and arthritis, coupled with the cold weather, she had greater difficulty getting there. She needed assistance to safely manage the stairs from her apartment, and now doubted her ability to get safely in and out of the bathtub. She wanted to live with one of her children or grandchildren but didn't think this was realistic because their lives were so busy. She described her own experience working with her sisters to care for her parents, and her frustration and disappointment that her children didn't do the same. She sometimes wished she had had a daughter, who she imagined would be a more devoted caregiver.

Geneva described her increasing problem with "nerves" and her racing heart, which caused her to worry that she'd have a heart attack while alone in her apartment. It was at these times she would go to the ER and was relieved to have been given the Xanax. When the psychiatrist told her it could be addictive, she was surprised, but also volunteered that she had taken more than prescribed because it helped her more.

Further inquiry about her symptoms found that, in addition to the anxiety symptoms noted in the consultation referral, Geneva had trouble falling and staying asleep and disinterest in eating. She felt fatigued, lethargic, amotivated, sad, and worthless much of the time, and had become a "cry-baby." She scored 19/30 on the GDS (moderately depressed) and 24/30 on MMSE (within normal range for her age and educational background). She did not appear to have signs of dementia. She said that she had never in her past felt so anxious or depressed.

Conceptualization

Geneva developed dependence on the anxiolytic medication and is experiencing comorbid anxiety and depression. Her presentation is consistent with major depression and generalized anxiety disorder with panic secondary to her medical condition. The depressive symptoms had not been noted in the ER. Her symptoms of anxiety and depression likely influenced each other–the anxiety symptoms made her feel increasingly helpless and hopeless, and the depressive symptoms made her feel less able to cope with her medical conditions and related anxiety.

Geneva has a long history of coping well with losses and transitions: Her husband's and son's deaths were buffered by the support of family and church, and her son's move had been tolerable given the support of her friends and church. However, her recent health problems, in combination with separation from family and loss of several friends, have contributed to her current difficulties.

Thoughts of living alone while feeling increasingly frail appeared to cause waves of anxiety, which at times escalated to feelings of panic when her cardiac symptoms were exacerbated. Feeling alone and scared contributed to increased depressive thoughts that she was not loved or worthy, which was clearly not true. The Xanax provided her with short-term relief, but could not address her underlying depression and social and residential concerns, and ultimately contributed to her injury and hospitalization.

Treatment

During her inpatient medical stay, the psychiatrist tapered Geneva off the Xanax and started her on an antidepressant (sertraline 50 mg), in combination with a low dose of a longer-acting anxiolytic medication (clonazepam 0.5 mg at bedtime) in the hopes of discontinuing the latter as the sertraline (Zoloft) became effective over the next four weeks.

After initial recovery from her hip surgery, Geneva was discharged to a subacute rehabilitation hospital. In this setting, she was seen again by a psychiatrist, who increased her Zoloft to 100 mg and discontinued the clonazepam, as well as by a psychologist and social worker. In individual treatment, the psychologist provided Geneva with education about rebound anxiety, which she had experienced from Xanax withdrawal, as well as anxiety reduction strategies (slow breathing, visualization). Further, they worked to understand the precipitants to Geneva's experience of panic, which were thoughts of being alone and separate from her family.

Together, Geneva and the psychologist worked with the social worker to develop plans for her discharge. Geneva's grandson, Titus, and his wife, Linda, attended a team meeting with the rehab physician, physical therapist, social worker, and psychologist. During the meeting, it became clear that family rules dictated that Geneva should be invited to live with Titus and Linda, but that Titus was reluctant to have his grandmother in their home. For months, Linda had been encouraging him to invite Geneva, but he hadn't. He was concerned about his grandmother's privacy: All the bedrooms and the bathroom were located upstairs in the small house. The living room could easily accommodate a daybed and dresser, but he was unsure if his grandma would be comfortable with this lack of privacy. Titus also wondered how she would be able to use the bathroom.

Geneva looked relieved and said to Titus, "I don't care about that. All I care about is being with my family." Brief problem-solving among the family resolved that a commode chair could be hidden with a screen, and she could have at least weekly baths with her granddaughter's help getting up the stairs and into and out of the bath. All agreed it wasn't ideal, but functional. Given Geneva's recovery and progress during physical therapy, a reasonable longer-term goal was for Geneva to climb the six stairs using a cane. The team also suggested an occupational therapy home evaluation (e.g., to recommend safety features for the bathroom) and made this referral.

Geneva's depression and anxiety were much improved in her new home. She was still able to attend church on Sundays, with rides from her family or from church members. Her granddaughter accompanied her to the follow-up primary care appointment and helped Geneva to explain the events of the prior few months. The primary doctor agreed she would help to monitor Geneva's depression and anxiety. She also encouraged Geneva and her family to call the clinic's on-call nurse whenever they were concerned about her breathing or other symptoms.

Comment

Older adults who present with prominent symptoms of anxiety should be assessed for depression, and vice versa, given that these problems so frequently co-occur. Geneva's situation is not uncommon, particularly for older women with multiple physical problems and/or interpersonal losses. Her situation is also not uncommon in that she did not have well-coordinated medical care. Though she did have a primary care doctor, she instead was receiving treatment in the ER (because of its proximity and immediate availability when she was frightened). Frequent ER visits can be suggestive of an anxiety disorder. Ideally, Geneva might have been referred back to her primary doctor and/or a mental health professional when her symptoms were first recognized. Further, she appeared to have trouble managing her symptoms of congestive heart failure. This issue, certainly both a cause of and exacerbated by the anxiety, might have been better addressed.

In addition to concern about multiple medical problems, Geneva's depression and anxiety were closely related to her unfulfilled expectation that her family should be taking closer care of her. Older adults differ–based on cultural and socioeconomic factors, as well as particular family relationships and personal preferences–in their desire to live alone, with family, or in other residential/nursing care environments. In Geneva's case, there was a clash between cultural norms and generational differences; ultimately, the cultural norms for filial (or grandfilial) responsibility were stronger than her grandson's practical or lifestyle concerns for her. If her family had not been able to take her in, the rehabilitation care team might have worked with her to consider home health aide services at home (e.g., to help her with baths) and/or a move to an assisted living facility. However, access to such services differs from locality to locality and options are often limited by financial constraints.

CHAPTER ELEVEN

Vascular Depression: George Marino

Older adults with cerebrovascular disease appear to be at relatively high risk for depression. Likewise, individuals who develop depression for the first time in late life are more likely to have evidence of structural and functional brain changes (e.g., on MRI studies and neuropsychological testing). Older adults with vascular disease or risk factors–including a history of stroke or heart attack, angina, hypertension, high cholesterol, or evidence of blocked arteries–may develop depression that is characterized by psychomotor retardation, poor motivation or initiative, poor insight, and relatively little guilt or other depressive ideation (Alexopoulos et al., 1997).

George's case demonstrates that vascular depression, along with changes in executive cognitive functions that often accompany the condition, can be challenging to treat and it highlights the importance of educating and eliciting support from families (Alexopoulos et al., 2000; Kalayam and Alexopoulos, 1999). And, because George suffered a severe stroke and did not survive, his case serves as a reminder that it is not uncommon for older, chronically ill patients to die in the midst of mental health treatment.

George Marino: Introduction

George, a 74-year-old Italian-American, married, retired insurance salesman, had multiple chronic medical problems over the past 10 years, including insulin-dependent diabetes and coronary artery disease. His heart bypass operation four years ago finally motivated him to quit drinking and smoking but he was still overweight, and although his doctor advised him to start walking for exercise, he just couldn't seem to get motivated. Not only wasn't he walking, but he mostly just sat and watched TV, whereas in the past he'd been so attentive to any necessary household repair that a burnt-out lightbulb wouldn't remain unreplaced for an hour. His wife, Rose, now nagged him to get anything done, and things were going from bad to worse between them. They had grown distant since he started having erectile problems five or six years ago; he was embarrassed and avoided contact with her. Lately, she was yelling at him all the time for being "lazy" and "useless."

When, during his annual exam, George's cardiologist asked him how things were going, George said he was feeling useless. Further questioning elicited that George was not enjoying much, was not motivated for usual activity, and felt worthless because of Rose's constant criticism of his laziness and her disappointment that he was no longer interested in sex. Although George said he was taking his prescribed medications every day, he admitted he wasn't paying careful attention to his diabetes management—he didn't always check his sugars and often ate too much. He had put on 10 pounds since their last visit.

The cardiologist explained that George's sexual problems could be related to his vascular disease and diabetes and/or possibly the medications he was taking. They had changed one of his blood pressure medications a few years ago because of sexual side effects, but this did not seem to help. George agreed to a urology referral for further evaluation. The cardiologist also suggested that George start on an antidepressant medication (sertraline), and offered to refer him to the psychologist for further evaluation of depression and possible help for George and his wife. George wanted to include Rose in the decisionmaking, so he invited her in from the waiting room. Rose said it was about time someone else noticed there was a problem, and they both agreed to the psychology referral.

Issues for Consideration

In cases like George's, it can be difficult to sort out the causes of observable behavioral changes. What are the relative and interacting influences of medical, cognitive, psychological, and interpersonal issues on his seemingly "lazy" and apathetic attitude? Certainly, his poorly managed diabetes, weight gain, and lack of exercise could contribute to poor energy or fatigue. Neurologically based cognitive changes can affect motivation, initiative, and even personality; depression can cause or exacerbate these same problems. Relationship stress can contribute to changes in self-esteem and communication, while depression can place stress on a relationship. A multifaceted evaluation can help to sort this out.

The impact of physical and behavioral changes on a couple's relationship can be significant, and the resulting relationship stress can then exacerbate behavioral problems. For example, George and his wife appeared to experience the unfortunate and common behavior pattern that occurs when a man develops erectile dysfunction: He is avoidant, she feels rejected and hurt, she becomes critical, and he further distances. Additionally, Rose's anger at George may, in part, relate to her misattributing his behavior changes to his character rather than to his medical, psychiatric, and/or neurological problems. The evaluation should address each of their attributions for George's problems.

Assessment

George and Rose met with the psychologist for an initial evaluation. They came 45 minutes early, as requested, to fill out some questionnaires (a brief medical and social history, the Geriatric Depression Scale, and a marital satisfaction questionnaire). During the meeting, George was relatively quiet, offering little spontaneously but responding appropriately to direct questions, although occasionally his replies were somewhat tangential. He tended to defer to Rose, who was emotionally reactive, talkative, and indirectly expressive of anger at George. She said that she had lost most of what felt good in their relationship. They used to enjoy sex, and now he didn't even seem to notice her. She used to count on him to help keep their home in such good repair, as well as to help cook on Sundays, and now he didn't seem to care. She complained that he kept breaking his promises, telling her constantly that he'd get to this project or that project later, but never getting around to it.

On the Mutuality Scale (Archbold et al., 1992), a brief questionnaire about relationship satisfaction, they both endorsed shared values on the positive side, but also both endorsed low shared pleasure, low affective closeness, and low reciprocity (i.e., mutual give-and-take); they further agreed there was sexual dissatisfaction and frequent yelling in their relationship but no physical violence or threats.

George said he couldn't really explain why he no longer felt motivated to help around the house. He did admit to feeling ashamed of his erectile dysfunction, saying that the problem wasn't that he didn't care for Rose, but that he felt he could no longer satisfy her. Rose too said she couldn't explain his behavior, but overall felt he didn't love her as much, as he didn't seem to put any effort toward trying to please her by helping at home and didn't show her affection. She couldn't understand why he would eventually do some chores when she nagged him, but not if she asked him politely in the morning and never on his own initiative.

The only activity that both George and Rose said they enjoyed together was visits with their three children and their spouses, and their eight grandchildren, all of whom lived in the area. Rose also enjoyed playing cards and shopping with her girlfriends, and attending church. George said he no longer had the interest for church, although sometimes Rose "demanded" that he go. He watched CNN and played word-find puzzles most of the day. He had retired nine years earlier, and missed having something to get up and do in the morning. Though he used to walk daily and work in the garden, he rarely felt up to doing either these days.

On the GDS, George scored 12 of 30 points, endorsing items including feeling bored, helpless, worthless, having dropped activities, starting but not finishing activities, and having trouble concentrating and making decisions. When questioned further, he reported adequate sleep and appetite, but acknowledged having passive suicidal thoughts (e.g., that he'd be better off dead since lately he felt so useless) with no plan of action and no history of suicidal intent. Rose scored 8 of 30 points on the GDS, endorsing items including worry about the future, getting upset over little things, feeling helpless, having trouble concentrating, and not feeling in good spirits most of the time. She also reported having trouble falling and staying asleep and worrying much of the time. She had no thoughts of suicide. Neither George nor Rose used alcohol and Rose took no psychotropic medications.

On a brief cognitive screening (3MS and clock drawing), George had trouble with a working memory task (could not spell "world" backward), verbal fluency (i.e., named four 4-legged animals in 30 seconds), and verbal recall (1 of 3 words after brief delay, recognized the other 2 from a choice; same pattern after longer delay) (3MS score = 83/100; MMSE = 25/30). The scores were somewhat lower than expected for his age and 14 years of education. Additionally, he had some trouble organizing his drawing of a clock (i.e., unable to set the hands to indicate the instructed time).

The psychologist told them that couple's therapy would likely help each of them to understand the other and interact more constructively together. She also referred George for a neuropsychological evaluation to help clarify his cognitive strengths and weaknesses. These test results, combined with an MRI scan of his brain that had been ordered, were available after the couple had attended several couple's sessions. The MRI suggested that George had significant subcortical microvascular disease. The neuropsychological evaluation confirmed the screening results, showing mild verbal recall and executive functioning deficits, that is, trouble in planning, organizing, and sequencing his responses to complex problems.

The psychologist also obtained George's permission to obtain a report from the urologist, which showed that George did have disrupted blood flow to the penis. He was offered several options to help him obtain and maintain an erection; according to the report, George decided to try the vacuum pump. He had inquired about sildenafil (Viagra), but his cardiac illness was a contraindication for trying it.

Conceptualization

George's case is complex but, unfortunately, not uncommon. He has symptoms of depression, some of which overlap with symptoms common to frontal brain changes, that is, decreased initiative, sense of apathy, and emotional flatness. The difficulty he has starting and following through with activities may reflect depression; his mood and behavioral changes may also be organically based. Working with George to stabilize his medical health—diabetes management, weight, exercise—might help to prevent further physical and cognitive decline.

Rose appears to be suffering from mild anxiety and depression. Her worry about George and their relationship is affecting her sleep, mood, concentration, and sense of control. Helping her to gain an increased understanding of George's condition, and thus an increased sense of control and likely less anger, will be important.

Marital issues are important for both George and Rose, as each is feeling rejected by and angry in interaction with the other. If Rose can be helped to have more realistic expectations and more accurate attributions for her husband's problems, she may not feel as disappointed and angered by his apparent disinterest. She also could be helped to understand that George can do more when he has structure and cues to guide him. She may need to take a more active role—in supervising his activity at home, as well as by initiating affectionate contact. Both had valued their sexual relationship and were missing it, and could be helped to renew their intimacy with some adaptations (Zeiss and Zeiss, 1999; Zeiss, Zeiss, and Davies, 1999).

Treatment

George and Rose agreed to continue biweekly couple's psychotherapy, while George's response to the antidepressant medication would continue to be monitored every few months by his regular primary care physician in consultation with a local psychiatrist; he did show some improvement in his mood and energy in the first month of taking the medication. Couple's sessions focused in three main areas: education, communication and mutual understanding, and grief regarding loss of George's previous abilities.

The psychologist provided education to the couple about depression, cerebrovascular disease, brain changes and their impact on George's behavior, sexuality, and behavioral health. She also gave them information about loss and grief, as the changes in George were losses for each of them. Although some of the changes may reverse as his depression improved, other changes would be enduring and less likely to change (e.g., his decreased ability to initiate activity).

The psychologist also recommended that the couple attend the clinic's diabetes education class, and emphasized that Rose would need to take a more active role in helping George to manage his diabetes and other medical problems. As he was having difficulty motivating himself to administer his daily glucose tests, and was not consistently taking his insulin and other medications, George agreed that Rose could supervise these aspects of his care. In addition, Rose admitted that she herself could use more exercise, and they agreed to walk together several mornings each week. Without Rose's own motivation, this would have been quite difficult.

Both George and Rose were feeling hurt by the other's behaviors—George by Rose's constant criticism of him, and Rose by George's apparent disinterest in her or their home. Rose was encouraged to change the tone of her "nagging." While her nagging had actually provided the structure and cuing George needed to get things done, she practiced cuing and instructing him with less anger. Her ability to make simple requests, rather than voicing criticism, helped George feel less worthless. George agreed that he missed physical intimacy with his wife, as she did with him. Rose reassured him that she didn't care that much about his erections but, if he wanted, she'd be willing for them to try the vacuum pump. Given George's generally poor motivation, Rose would need to learn to initiate intimate contact, which was new and difficult for her. They were both helped by the reassurance that each still cared for the other.

Between sessions, Rose was working to practice clear, but uncritical, communication with George, as well as trying to initiate hugs and kisses with him. Realizing that she could no longer "wait for him to notice" a home repair problem, or remember her request from the day before, she was instead asking him to help with a problem when she wanted it done. She also realized that some tasks were now too complicated for him to complete on his own, and they needed to ask for assistance from their sons. Both George and Rose found it difficult to accept these changes, and were sad about the losses, but they were slowly managing to adapt with the new skills they had learned.

After three months—or six meetings—Rose left a message for the psychologist that they couldn't make their next session. George had been taken by ambulance to the hospital for what seemed to be a major stroke; he was unconscious in the ICU. Two days later, Rose called to say he had died from a massive cerebral hemorrhage. A month later, after the funeral and the out-of-town visitors had left, Rose returned to the psychologist. She was grieving, and feeling guilty about her prior anger and criticism of her husband. However, she also spoke of feeling grateful that their last month together had been less conflictual and more affectionate. Rose received a lot of support now from her sister, children, and girlfriends, and knew it would take time for her to grieve. The psychologist told Rose she could return at any time if she was feeling concerned about her level of distress or her ability to function at home.

Comment

Though vascular depression is not a formal diagnostic entity at this time, it appears to capture a syndrome of mood and motivational change common among older adults with vascular brain disease. It is potentially responsive to antidepressant medication, but intervention for such patients should also include efforts to increase structure, supervision, and support for engaging in healthy behaviors and enjoyable activities. In general, geriatric mental health care often entails working to sort out which affective, cognitive, or behavioral changes in an older adult can be reversed, to help optimize the older adult's functioning using existing personal strengths and interpersonal and environmental resources, and to grieve and accept losses that cannot be changed.

George and Rose had many strengths–long-standing affection, a previously good sexual relationship, her motivation and willingness to participate in treatment and change her behavior–that helped them to adjust to difficult challenges in late life. In contrast, couples with long-standing conflict and anger and/or significant health or cognitive changes in both individuals will have a poorer prognosis for adapting to late-life changes.

As was true for this couple, sexuality remains an important part of living for older adults (Hillman, 2000), and aging-related physical changes, illness, or psychiatric problems can negatively affect sexual functioning. In working with older couples, it is important to remember that their beliefs about "appropriate" sexual behavior and/or gender roles in the sexual relationship may be relatively traditional. In this case, Rose had rarely, if ever, been the initiator of sexual contact in their relationship. If either partner has problems that interfere with intercourse, many older couples can be comfortable with alternatives to intercourse for sexual stimulation if education and reassurance are provided.

A Note About Death and Dying

George's death was an abrupt loss–to his family and to his professional caregivers. He obviously had many risk factors for stroke, but had seemed stable and appeared to be making progress in several areas. One difficult aspect of working with older adults is that we are confronted with death and dying. This reality challenges us to face fears about mortality in ourselves and in our loved ones. It also provides a rich opportunity to talk with older patients about end-of-life concerns, advance care planning (e.g., completing advance directives, making funeral arrangements), and life review issues.

An important adult developmental point to keep in mind is that, by the time adults reach their seventies or eighties, they are typically accepting of their eventual death, yet are frequently concerned about how they might die (e.g., about being a burden to their loved ones). Older adults are often more comfortable discussing issues of death and dying than are their young or middle-aged doctors or therapists. In settings where death is commonplace (e.g., long-term care nursing homes), professionals should be aware of the impact of frequent loss on both caregiving staff and other patients receiving care. Programs that offer both remembrance for the deceased and bereavement support for the survivors are helpful in these settings.

CHAPTER TWELVE

Dementia and Depression: Olga and Sven Thompson

Increasing age is the primary risk factor for developing a dementing illness (such as Alzheimer's disease, vascular dementia, or dementia secondary to Parkinson's disease). The afflicted proportion of the population rises from 6–8% of adults over the age of 65 to approximately 30% of those over the age of 85 (Small et al., 1997). Dementia refers to a constellation of memory and other cognitive deficits that result in declines in an individual's ability to function independently and it often occurs with disorders of mood and disturbances of behavior, including depression, anxiety, agitation, or delusions. Conversely, cognitive deficits—which may or may not relate to an underlying dementia—are frequently among the symptoms presented by depressed older adults (Storandt and VandenBos, 1995).

For example, does a disheveled older woman who has stopped playing cards, reading novels, and cooking, and who has trouble telling her history in a clear and coherent manner, suffer from depression, dementia, both, or something else entirely?[1] Collaboration with a geriatrician, geriatric psychiatrist, neurologist, geropsychologist, and/or neuropsychologist is often required to help sort out these difficult diagnostic questions. Further, providing education, support, and referral as needed to family caregivers, who are themselves at high risk for depression and exhaustion, is critical (Zarit, 1996).

Olga and Sven Thompson: Introduction

Sven and Olga Thompson, both in their late seventies, had been married for 52 years. Both were retired teachers; he had taught and coached high school and she had taught elementary school. Olga was diagnosed with Alzheimer's disease about one year ago. That evaluation and diagnosis were precipitated by Sven's realization that something must be wrong with her—over the period of a few years, she became increasingly forgetful, asked questions repeatedly, was easily confused in the kitchen, needed reminders to shower, and was uncharacteristically needy and clinging. Sven had taken over most responsibilities at home, and gradually was becoming Olga's primary caregiver. He was feeling tired, frustrated, sad, lonely, and was ashamed for losing his temper so frequently. Sven responded to an advertisement in the local paper recruiting participants for a research treatment study of support groups for early-stage dementia (Yale, 1995) and for dementia caregivers (Gallagher-Thompson and DeVries, 1994). After a brief telephone screening, they were invited in for an evaluation.

Issues for Consideration

A caregiver's understanding of dementia—Is the person viewed as "lazy" or as incapable of prior behaviors?—will affect how that caregiver copes with the illness. In the case of Sven and Olga, how does that understanding affect their relationship? The behavioral changes that come with Alzheimer's disease can be particularly hard to accept because the person usually looks quite healthy and can maintain pleasant social skills. The threat of losing an accustomed relationship with a spouse or a parent, together with fears for the future, can sometimes lead families to deny that a problem exists until deficits become so severe that they undermine the patient's safety. Shifting power balances in families—that is, changes in who has responsibility for and control over what—create additional stress when an older family member is sick, placing particular strain on relationships between parents and adult children (Qualls, 1999).

In addition to the cognitive deficits of dementia, we must examine the impact of secondary disturbances on both the demented person's behavior and the caregiver's capacity to cope. Depression in the patient can exaggerate functional deficits in dementia, making the burden of care even heavier. And, depression in the caregiver–related to feeling exhausted, irritable, helpless, hopeless–can cause very real limitations in the ability to manage the demands of caregiving along with taking care of oneself. Caregivers, as well as individuals with dementia, should always be screened for depression.

Many family caregivers are reluctant to ask for help with their situation or do not know whom to approach or how. Accordingly, educating families about community resources is central to working with them. Different cultural groups perceive both the burden of and responsibility for caregiving differently and different norms govern their use of formal support services and nursing homes. Likewise, different individuals, especially spouses, may feel responsible to care for their relative on their own, perhaps as a sign of loyalty and love or perhaps as a signal of their discomfort in exposing to others how "strange" their loved one has become. Sven's response to an advertisement suggests that he was indeed ready to look for or accept help. He may or may not require additional services to help care for Olga at home, depending on his own level of physical, cognitive, and emotional functioning, and on his access to practical and emotional support from family and friends.

Assessment

During intake evaluations for the group programs, Sven and Olga each completed individual interviews and a brief assessment battery. Olga was attentive, pleasant, and verbal, but had difficulty relating her history with any depth or specificity. On a brief mental status screen (Modified Mini-Mental State Exam, or 3MS, and a clock drawing test), she demonstrated good attention and language comprehension and expression skills but was disoriented to time and had significant short-term memory problems (she could not recall or recognize three words after a brief delay) and executive functioning deficits (difficulty with verbal fluency and clock drawing); her MMSE score was 22/30 and her 3MS score was 71/100. On the Geriatric Depression Scale

(16/30), she reported moderate symptoms of depression, including sad mood, worry, helplessness, loss of interest, not feeling happy, worthlessness, and feeling like crying.

When asked how things were at home, she became tearful and said that she thought Sven was angry with her, saying, "He is so critical, and he gets so uptight all the time. I can't seem to do anything right." Olga did have some insight into the fact that her memory was impaired and knew she had the diagnosis of Alzheimer's disease, and said she felt ashamed about making so many mistakes.

On intake, Sven discussed—tearfully at times—his frustration and feelings of helplessness with his wife. He knew she was sick but kept hoping that, if he tried to encourage her, she might be able to cook and do other chores as she had before. But despite his efforts, she kept failing miserably and his irritation increased. He was ashamed for yelling at her sometimes.

The interview, together with his scores on the Beck Depression Inventory-II (BDI-II = 21), Beck Anxiety Inventory (BAI = 24), and Modified Mini-Mental State Exam (3MS = 96/100), revealed that he was cognitively intact but with symptoms of a major depressive disorder and generalized anxiety disorder. He reported fatigue, little energy or motivation or interest in things, and consistent sleep disruption, worry and fear, and somatic problems, including dizziness, indigestion, wobbly legs, and inability to relax. His general health was otherwise good except for hypertension that was being managed by medication. He said he had no thoughts of suicide or of harming his wife, but he was upset by how much he was criticizing her. Afraid to leave Olga alone and embarrassed to bring her for social outings, he had stopped most usual contact with their friends. And, believing that his three children, who lived within one hour's drive, were too busy with their own lives and families, he seldom asked for their help.

Sven also completed the Revised Memory and Behavior Problems Checklist (Teri et al., 1992) to indicate how frequently Olga evidenced certain difficult behaviors and how upsetting he found each behavior to be. According to Sven, she demonstrated the following problems at least three to six times in the past week: asking the same question over and over, trouble remembering recent events, losing or misplacing things, forgetting what day it is, starting but not finishing things, difficulty concentrating on a task, appearing anxious or worried, appearing sad or depressed, expressing feelings of hopelessness or sadness about the future, and comments about feeling worthless or being a burden to others. He indicated that most of these behaviors upset him "very much."

Conceptualization

Both Olga and Sven were excellent candidates for their respective skills-based support group interventions. Both had medical care attended to by their primary care physician and records were obtained documenting prior workup of Olga's dementia. Both of them met criteria for major depression; neither expressed suicidal ideation nor other imminent risk issues. Both were dealing with changes in their relationship to each other, changes in their self-perceptions, and changes in their relationships with family and friends. Olga was verbal, had some insight into her deficits, had appropriate interpersonal skills, and would fit well into the early dementia support group. Sven, who was motivated for treatment, needed education about Alzheimer's disease and about more appropriate strategies for communicating with Olga, as well as for managing his frustration and learning to ask for help so he could take an occasional break.

Treatment

Dementia and caregiver skills-building classes were structured as an eight-week intervention, with booster sessions at one month and two months after the weekly classes had completed. Each session was two hours long, typically with a break after 45–50 minutes. Individuals with dementia and their caregivers did not interact during the class sessions.

Sven participated in caregiver skills-based training, which included education about the cognitive changes caused by dementia and introduced both cognitive coping skills (i.e., understanding how thoughts influence feelings, identifying dysfunctional thought patterns) and behavioral skills (relaxation, assertive communication) and their application to situations that were causing him excessive anger and guilt. Through this intervention, Sven was able to shift to more realistic expectations of Olga; as he became more accepting of her diagnosis and what it meant for her day-to-day functioning, his critical comments decreased. And, as Sven became less tense and angry and started to take some time off for himself with the help of his daughters, Olga's mood also improved and she appeared less clinging and frightened.

Olga was active in her group meetings, and was relieved to talk, in an atmosphere of patience and structure, with others who were also recently diagnosed with dementia. The group leader provided education about dementia and related family and legal issues (e.g., power of attorney). Group members discussed their experiences coping with the illness, the reactions from family and friends, and their feelings of loss. They practiced relaxation exercises, which Olga particularly enjoyed.

By the end of the eight weeks, Olga no longer met criteria for depression but Sven had persisting mild depression (BDI-II = 15), including disrupted sleep. He was referred for an antidepressant medication evaluation and continued individual outpatient psychotherapy to reinforce new skills for managing his combined depression, grief, anger, and anxiety. During these sessions, Sven was able to leave Olga at home with a paid assistant arranged through the local department of senior services.

Six months later, Olga's condition had declined to the extent that she needed more personal care than Sven felt he could provide. Sven was able to discuss the problem with Olga and their children, who agreed that a joint move to an assisted living facility where she could receive daily help would be in Olga's best interest; and nursing home care was available at the same site should her progressive illness require it.

Comment

This case illustrates how treating depression in a caregiver can help the behavior of the person with dementia. Likewise, treating depression in dementia can ameliorate depressive symptoms in the caregiver (Teri et al., 1997). Support groups offered concurrently for individuals with dementia and their caregivers constitute an ideal care model because lack of supervision for the patient is a common barrier to caregiver attendance; it remains difficult to fund, however, and is not available in most settings. Nonetheless, treating depression in individuals with dementia and their caregivers is an important source of hope for improved functioning and lessened despair.

Note

1. Note that cognitive changes in late life range from mild changes common to normal aging to more severe deficits resulting from disease. Here is a brief summary of causes of cognitive change:

- *Normal aging:* With advancing age, it is normal to have more trouble retrieving information, finding the right words, manipulating information mentally, or solving problems as quickly. Memory aids such as calendars and reducing distractions and anxiety can help.
- *Acute mental status changes/delirium:* Sudden changes in mental status, such as poor or shifting attention and confusion or disorientation, usually reflect delirium caused by a medical problem or medication reaction. Such acute mental status changes indicate need for immediate medical attention to rule out an infection, toxic reaction, dehydration, or other acute problem.
- *Dementia:* Dementia entails a constellation of cognitive deficits that cause significant impairment in social or occupational functioning and include memory impairment (trouble learning new information or recalling previously learned information) plus one or more of the following: aphasia (language disturbance), apraxia (impaired ability to carry out motor activities, e.g., getting dressed), agnosia (inability to recognize or identify objects despite intact sensory function), or executive functioning deficits (trouble planning, organizing, sequencing, abstracting). The pattern and course of cognitive deficits over time vary depending on the type of dementing illness.

- *Focal deficits:* Specific cognitive deficits that may not meet criteria for dementia (e.g., changes in language or visual-perceptual functioning) may result from stroke or other cerebrovascular disease.
- *Cognitive deficits secondary to psychiatric illness:* Depression, anxiety, and alcohol abuse can cause problems with concentration, memory, and problem-solving that can be reversed with treatment of the psychiatric illness. Long-standing alcohol abuse or dependence can cause irreversible cognitive deficits.

CHAPTER THIRTEEN

Alcohol Abuse and Depression: Dave Gilbert

Although younger adults are more likely to suffer from alcohol abuse or dependence than their elders, at-risk drinking remains a significant health and mental health problem for older adults (Center for Substance Abuse Treatment, 1998). Older adults who consume too much alcohol can suffer from disorientation, memory problems, falls, sleep trouble, poor nutrition, mood changes, and poor self-care (Barry and Blow, 1999). Depressed older adults are at higher risk for alcohol misuse, and the reverse is also true—that is, alcohol use can exacerbate symptoms of depression. Therefore, screening for alcohol and other substance abuse is a vital component of the mental health evaluation. Dave's case illustrates how a relapse of alcohol abuse during a stressful time led to increased depression and suicidality. Treatment of the alcohol abuse was central to his care.

Dave Gilbert: Introduction

Dave Gilbert, a healthy, active, and sociable 76-year-old veteran (World War II, Navy, minimal combat exposure, no history of posttraumatic stress disorder) and retired housepainter, was having a difficult time maintaining his usual optimism. His marriage to Betsy had always been difficult, but lately he was losing his temper more often than not and having trouble sleeping. A year ago, his VA primary care doctor had given him lorazepam (Ativan) to help him relax and sleep at night. He had also been referred to an older men's support group, where he attended weekly meetings run by a psychologist. In that setting, he learned strategies to cope with stress and manage his anger.

In the group, it also became clear from Dave's description that his wife was suffering cognitive changes and he was encouraged to take her for a dementia evaluation. The evaluation suggested that Betsy had vascular dementia with mild changes in her memory and initiative. Dave and Betsy attended several meetings with the psychologist after her diagnosis to discuss strategies to help them both adjust to changes in her abilities. With these interventions, Dave managed relatively well for the next few months.

In recent weeks, however, Dave had missed several group meetings and, when he attended, he was uncharacteristically tearful and subdued. He shared that he did not feel like himself and didn't feel he could tolerate the stress at home any longer; marital conflict, his wife's continued decline, and recent financial stressors were all taking a toll on him. He did not consider divorce as an option for practical and moral reasons; his wife increasingly depended on him to take care of her and the house. With continued discussion, he admitted that he was drinking again—a couple of beers at the VFW post in the afternoon, and a screwdriver at home at night. Dave had a history of heavy drinking—one of many problems for the marriage—but had been sober during the 15 years since his heart attack. He said he started drinking about a month ago because it helped him to relax and sleep, and he did not view his current drinking as excessive or harmful.

In his initial report, he minimized both the amount he consumed and the impact it was having on his mood and functioning; when asked specifically to describe recent consumption, he admitted to three beers in the afternoon and three screwdrivers at night. In addition, during a follow-up couple's session, Dave's wife said she knew he was drinking again because she could see it in his eyes and his actions; she said his irritability and temper were worse when he was drinking.

During group meetings, he discussed feelings of depression and hopelessness about his marital conflict, but said he had no thoughts, plan, or intent to harm himself or his wife. Still, assessing Dave's suicide risk was critical. There was no history of suicidal thoughts or behavior, major depression, or physical violence in the relationship. An avid hunter for years, he did have guns at home, and he insisted that he felt safe to keep them. He was able to discuss a plan he would undertake if he felt more hopeless or unsafe, namely, to contact the hospital emergency services.

Many of the group members were encouraging Dave to stop drinking, and he conceded that he should try to cut down. He had accepted a referral to a psychiatrist for evaluation of his depression, and was advised to taper off the Ativan and start on sertraline (Zoloft). Within several weeks, however, Dave presented to the emergency room stating that he was scared by suicidal thoughts of crashing his car.

Issues for Consideration

This case highlights the importance of ongoing assessment during the course of treatment. When an older patient has a substance abuse history, it is important to be aware of risks for and signs of relapse. Any notable change in the person's mood, functioning, or mental status should raise the question. Dave had become more withdrawn in the group setting—a warning sign given his usually outgoing and optimistic personality. Like most problem drinkers, he minimized his drinking and its potentially negative impact. Note that an excess of two drinks daily for older men (and one daily for women) is considered at-risk drinking (Adams, Barry, and Fleming, 1996). Specific questions about his use of alcohol elicited—although somewhat belatedly—the serious nature of his relapse.

This case also highlights the complex interaction between psychosocial stress, depression, alcohol use, and suicidal thoughts (Brennan and Moos, 1996). It can be difficult to sort out which problems came first—Did the increased stress of caregiving and the marital tension contribute to ineffective coping by drinking? Did the drinking cause increased stress and lead to depression?–and where treatment should focus (the depression symptoms? the alcohol use? the marital problems? the caregiving?). And, of course, safety is always the most immediate concern: Does Dave have a history of suicidal ideation or behavior? What resources does he have to cope with suicidal feelings?

Assessment

Assessment occurred over time in the context of ongoing mental health treatment. Recognition of his increased depression in a group treatment setting led to uncovering his relapsed alcohol abuse. And it was the surfacing of suicidal thoughts that brought him to Emergency Services at the VA Hospital, where the psychiatry triage staff felt that Dave would benefit from voluntary admission.

The precipitant for this crisis was his discovery of an urgent home repair that he could not afford. That night he drank excessively and felt very depressed. The next morning, on the way to the grocery store, he thought about driving off the road and then headed for the VA hospital instead.

The admitting psychiatrist did not suspect that Dave would require detoxification from his alcohol use; he had no withdrawal symptoms when he was not drinking. The psychiatrist asked Dave questions about his symptoms of depression and alcohol abuse, as well as current stressors and the history of his recent suicidal thinking. Dave spoke of anger at his wife's behaviors and his daughter Nancy's reneging on repaying money she owed to him. Dave admitted he had been having thoughts about suicide for the prior few weeks, because he was feeling helpless to manage the care of his wife with the constant conflict, but his sense of responsibility to his family kept him from acting on these thoughts.

However, when he realized he couldn't afford to fix the roof, he felt anxious and angry, started to drink, and felt more hopeless than ever. In the hospital, he expressed relief for being safe in the hospital, but otherwise felt helpless, hopeless, and worthless.

Conceptualization

Dave's multiple stressors had become overwhelming for him: his wife's decline, their long history of marital conflict, and financial problems. He had historically used alcohol to cope with strain at home; his relapse exacerbated his depressive symptoms and further impaired his ability to cope. A comprehensive treatment plan would need to: target his safety, depression, and alcohol relapse; evaluate and address family system issues, especially understanding the impact of his wife's vascular dementia; and help Dave improve strategies for managing ongoing stress.

Treatment

When Dave was admitted, he asked the team social worker to call his wife Betsy and daughter Nancy. Dave spoke to them and Nancy agreed to take the hour ride to bring Betsy to her home while Dave was in the hospital. Betsy and Nancy agreed to come in for a family meeting several days later.

Dave spoke with the social worker about the stresses at home; they agreed that, according to the "rules" of his family system, Dave was unable to ask for help with his wife or to stop rescuing his daughter from her financial problems. Dave acknowledged that his admission to the hospital was a way he chose to "shake up" the family system—by highlighting his need for help now that increasing depression and alcohol use had disabled his usually strong problem-solving capacities. Dave and the social worker identified several goals for the family meeting: for Dave to admit he was having drinking problems, to assert that he needed more help at home and to explore options, and to admit his financial limitations.

The psychiatrist reviewed Dave's medications with him. He was taking a blood pressure medication and a multivitamin. He had discontinued his outpatient Zoloft prescription after several days because it had caused him to have diarrhea, and he wasn't convinced he needed it. He had stopped taking the Ativan per the outpatient psychiatrist's advice. Dave was concerned about his trouble sleeping and his constant worrying and irritability. The psychiatrist recommended a trial of the antidepressant nefazodone (Serzone) to help with his sleep and depression.

The family meeting was attended by Dave, his wife and daughter, and the team psychiatrist, nurse, and social worker. Dave was able to admit that he felt overwhelmed at times by Betsy's declining abilities, which only made worse their long-standing bickering. Because she was afraid to be alone, and he was reluctant to leave her, he was leaving home only for necessary errands and had stopped his bowling and volunteering with the local veterans organization. The team discussed that both Dave and Betsy would benefit from "respite" provided by an adult day care program. Dave also needed further education about the memory and behavioral deficits of dementia so that he could have realistic expectations of Betsy; he was given reading materials and a contact number for a local dementia caregiver support group.

During the meeting, Dave expressed his upset at Nancy's financial troubles and not keeping her word to repay him what he had loaned her. He and Betsy lived on a fixed income and any unexpected expense—such as the recent roof repair—created an uncomfortable strain. Nancy had given him a check for part of the loan when she came to the hospital. She said it was a hardship but she didn't want him to be sick over it. This would help toward the roof repair.

Dave admitted to Betsy and Nancy that he had started to drink again and that he realized it made him feel worse rather than better. He agreed to attend a two-week day hospital substance abuse program followed by weekly relapse prevention therapy meetings.

Dave was discharged after one week, and started the day hospital program. There, veterans with recent substance abuse/dependence problems attended psychoeducational and therapy groups focused on relapse prevention. Dave worked to acknowledge the extent of his drinking problem and to identify alternative means of coping with anger, frustration, and stress. His exposure to other veterans with extremely serious consequences of their alcoholism—including homelessness, loss of careers, loss of relationships—was a "wake-up" call for him. As one of the oldest men in the program, he took on a paternal role and felt that he should be a positive role model for the younger men. This helped to motivate him to recommit to sobriety and to find constructive solutions to his problems.

Meanwhile, Dave's daughter brought Betsy to see her physician, who helped make referrals to a local low-income adult day care program that she could attend three days per week. When Dave completed the day hospital program, he began a 10-week individual relapse prevention therapy program, meeting 30 minutes per week with an alcohol counselor. He also returned to his weekly outpatient support group with the psychologist. He gave permission for the alcohol counselor and psychologist to talk as a way to facilitate coordination of his outpatient care. In the support group setting, he was open about his alcohol problems and treatment.

Six months after his hospitalization, he had not started drinking again. He reported improved ability to manage his anger and communicate effectively at home. He was working to accept that Betsy could no longer do all that she had previously done or control her memory problems. Realizing that he had to make time for some enjoyable relaxation during the week, he started bowling and volunteering again. He knew he needed to be alert for increased symptoms of depression or cravings to drink and was open to ongoing monitoring of these issues in the support group setting.

Comment

Dave was a highly motivated, intelligent, and personable individual who needed a fair amount of support to interrupt a potentially severe relapse of his alcohol abuse and related depression and suicidality. Treatment needed to address the substance abuse, depression, anger and stress management, family system issues, need for caregiver education and support, and services for his wife. In part, Dave's suicidal feelings were borne out of feeling a loss of control and a painful realization that he alone could not handle everything. With treatment, he realized that his ability to maintain optimism, solve problems, and manage his anger were better when he was not drinking, that he could help himself by taking advantage of services to help his wife, and that he felt better when he took some time to pursue pleasurable activities outside the home.

It is important to note that older adults who are abusing drugs or alcohol are not always best served through general substance abuse treatment programs. It is important in working with older adults to respect generational beliefs about alcohol use, to address age-related health and cognitive risks of alcohol use, and to use respectful and supportive rather than confrontational approaches to treatment (Center for Substance Abuse Treatment, 1998; Dupree and Schonfeld, 1999). Other important considerations are to collaborate with the elder's primary care physician in addressing health risks of alcohol use (Fleming et al., 1999), to address alcohol use as a critical barrier for treating depression, and to seek consultation with providers who have experience treating older substance abusers.

CHAPTER FOURTEEN

Personality Disorder and Depression: Dorothy Gleason

Personality disorders frequently persist into late life, although research regarding their relationship to aging remains in its infancy. There is a significant overlap between personality disorder and depression in older adults, as there is in younger ones (Zweig and Hillman, 1999). Older adults with personality disorders are more vulnerable to developing major depression, and these patients seem to be less responsive to treatments for depression (Gradman, Thompson, and Gallagher-Thompson, 1999). Delivering health care services to elders with personality disorders, particularly in institutional settings, can be stressful for patients and caregivers alike (Rosowsky et al., 1997). Dorothy's case illustrates depression onset in the context of health changes and temporary nursing home placement in a woman with narcissistic personality disorder. Helping nursing home staff to understand and respond constructively to her demanding behavior was an important part of treating Dorothy's depression (Rosowsky and Smyer, 1999).

Dorothy Gleason: Introduction

Dorothy Gleason was 84 and had been living alone since her second husband's death 15 years ago, shortly after which she was diagnosed with breast cancer and underwent a mastectomy. Aging in general was an appalling challenge for Dorothy, who had always been very conscientious about her body and liked to look just right. After her right breast removal, she felt that everyone knew that her body was defective. More recently, increasingly severe rheumatoid arthritis had disfigured her hands and required her to use a quad-cane for walking, both of which she found humiliating. In addition, she now had to worry about watching her diet because of her non-insulin-dependent diabetes.

Things went from bad to worse during the three-week period preceding her admission to a nursing home rehabilitation unit. First, she fell in the living room, causing a rug burn on her left elbow that developed into a skin ulcer she was unable to treat herself. The next week, she had a slight stroke that resulted in mild hemiparesis on her left side. She called her sister, who was her closest source of support, and was ultimately admitted to the rehab unit at the Oakdale Ridge Nursing Home. Dorothy had minimal contact with her son from her first marriage, which ended in divorce, and she had no other children.

Dorothy could not stand being surrounded by "decrepit old people" on the rehab unit. She avoided the other patients and, instead, spent time trying to forge relationships with nursing staff, to whom she voiced many criticisms about the feeble residents at Oakdale. Soon, she began criticizing the staff: No matter who provided her wound care, it was never thorough, timely, or caring enough and she tended to bad-mouth certain nurses when others were caring for her. Further, staff's attempts to reassure her that she was "lucky"—that her stroke was slight and she would likely have 90–95% recovery—infuriated her. She began isolating herself in her room and asking why God would want her to suffer endlessly in this useless and defective state.

Staff at the facility found Dorothy to be intolerable and demanding. She offered only negative and degrading comments about herself, her situation, the other residents, and the staff. The nurses and aides sought to avoid her as much as possible and argued at morning report about who would be stuck with Dorothy's care on a given day. Because the staff's avoidance confirmed Dorothy's beliefs that they were lazy and uncaring and that her life was miserable, she complained more and more that no one ever helped her or did their job. Finally the treatment team, disgusted with her behavior, asked the consulting psychologist to please evaluate and "fix" Dorothy.

Issues for Consideration

The relationship between depression and personality disorder can be difficult to sort out. Is Dorothy depressed? What is the impact of her apparent narcissistic personality disorder on her current adaptation? Also, what might be the impact of her stroke on cognitive, affective, or personality functioning? Are any of these issues affecting her ability to participate in her rehabilitation?

Although the transition from independent living to institutional care is almost universally a stressful one, varying personalities adapt quite differently. For example, individuals with dependent personality styles tend to have an easier time adjusting to life in a hospital or nursing home, as their reliance on others fits well with the demands of the setting. For Dorothy, what about her coping style is making her adjustment to a rehab nursing home stay so difficult? How do interactions between Dorothy and the staff affect her care and her adjustment?

Assessment

Dorothy agreed to participate in an interview with the consulting psychologist. She had little difficulty answering questions about herself and, although hostile in her tone, also appeared grateful that someone was listening to her complaints. She scored 92/100 on the 3MS, which is in the normal range for her age and high school education. (She had trouble copying intersecting pentagons, likely due to a combination of her stroke and rheumatoid arthritis.) On the Geriatric Depression Scale, she scored 23 of 30 points, suggesting that further evaluation of depression was important.

Dorothy told the psychologist that all her problems hinged on two things: having had a stroke that "couldn't be rehabilitated" and having to stay at Oakdale surrounded by feeble and senile residents and treated by lazy, rude, and incompetent staff. She also described her disgust with her body following the mastectomy and said that losing her breast was much more difficult than losing a husband of 48 years. Now expecting "only a 90–95% recovery" from a stroke, she felt even more damaged and imperfect.

Dorothy couldn't understand why God would let her continue living in such a wretched state. She was not able to accept the psychologist's observations that she could still do most things and instead voiced hopelessness about her future and doubts about the utility of rehabilitation when she was going to be crippled anyway. While denying active suicidal ideation, she said she wished often that God would take her. She reported experiencing no joy or happiness, even when her sister Martha visited. She couldn't concentrate on reading or television and no longer enjoyed eating; she wished the staff would stop badgering her about her food intake. She hated the mornings, because she hadn't been able to sleep past 4:00 A.M. since coming to Oakdale and felt just miserable. The last thing she felt like doing every morning at 10:00 were her exercises with the physical therapist.

The psychologist gave Dorothy feedback that she appeared to be experiencing a moderate depression, and that interactions between residents and long-term care staff can get complicated. The psychologist said she thought she could help, both by working individually with Dorothy to discuss the difficult changes she was experiencing and by working with the staff to help them with their interactions with Dorothy. She also told Dorothy that they could consider a psychiatric medication evaluation if these initial interventions did not help. Dorothy doubted that therapy could help her but was willing to talk to someone who was willing to listen to her, and also thought it would be great if the psychologist could "get those lazy nurses to do their jobs."

Conceptualization

Dorothy is a self-described perfectionist with an apparent narcissistic personality style that is accompanied by fairly inflexible thinking patterns (e.g., her belief that her body was entirely defective after her mastectomy, her belief that anything less than a full recovery from her stroke is worthless). Dorothy's self-focus was salient in her greater difficulty coping with her breast surgery than with her husband's death, about which the psychologist noted almost no evidence of sadness or grief.

On the basis of the interview, the GDS, and staff report, Dorothy has a moderate major depression that may have multiple determinants, including possible mood change secondary to her stroke, loss of control, and the threats to her self-esteem posed by physical changes and institutional care. In addition, because of her narcissistic personality style, she likely feels even more vulnerable in this setting. To compensate for her fears of increased disability and dependence, she is demanding and expects immediate validation of her concerns from staff, but her attempts to elicit it are backfiring. The nurses' avoidance increases her sense of isolation, vulnerability, and worthlessness, illustrating a pattern of interaction that requires a systemic approach to intervention.

Treatment

Treatment initially focused on two specific interventions: staff education and individual psychotherapy with Dorothy.

The psychologist met with the head nurse and was invited to attend afternoon report to gather more information about the staff's perceptions of and difficulties working with Dorothy. She heard their complaints about Dorothy "thinking of herself as the Queen Resident" and her demands and criticism of them and other residents. Contrary to their usual dedication to caring for sick elders, not one nurse or aide voiced sympathy for Dorothy's medical problems. The psychologist acknowledged that Dorothy had a very off-putting way of coping with feelings of insecurity and informed the staff that she also appeared to suffer from a major depression. The psychologist asked to return the following week to discuss ideas for helping both Dorothy and the staff.

During the next meeting, the psychologist helped staff to understand how typical interactions with Dorothy reflected the thoughts and feelings of the parties involved. For example, when approaching Dorothy for her wound change and hearing her haughty and indirect criticism—"Doesn't this wound look terrible? You'd better take your time with this dressing"—the nurses construed her as ungrateful and impossible to please and thus they would feel unappreciated and angry. In response, they tended to respond curtly or defensively, for example, "I'm moving as quickly as I can." The psychologist explained that, to Dorothy, this perceived rejection confirmed her belief that she was defective and uncared for. Hurt and angry, she continued to focus on the negative, pushing staff further away and fueling a nonproductive and vicious cycle.

The psychologist shared her own experience of working with Dorothy; she found her to have the potential to be charming in spite of her fairly bitter complaints because she was easily engaged to talk about herself and responded well to empathy about her experiences. The psychologist provided a brief description of narcissistic personality and how such individuals tend to require consistent attention and admiration to maintain their sense of esteem while having difficulty understanding the impact of their behaviors on others. She also acknowledged the staff division that can occur when the patient perceives certain staff to be more caring (such as the mental health professional who has more time to listen) and advised the nurses to take care not to reinforce this by venting frustration about each other when Dorothy started to complain.

Over the next few weeks, the nursing staff practiced communicating empathy rather than negativity in response to Dorothy's complaints (e.g., "This whole experience has been very difficult for you, hasn't it Mrs. Gleason?"). Per the psychologist's recommendation, they also tried to spend a consistent ten minutes with Dorothy during each wound change rather than rushing through it in five. The staff, initially skeptical, was surprised to see that, over time, Dorothy actually responded more positively when asked questions about herself, shown empathy, and given a little extra time.

Concurrent with this staff intervention, the psychologist met twice weekly with Dorothy for a month. The therapy sessions focused on educating Dorothy about the impact of her black-

and-white thinking style on her depression. Dorothy was able to identify the feelings of vulnerability and fear she experienced as her body and abilities were changing, and how this contributed to her beliefs that she was useless, hopeless, and unlovable. She gained some ability to understand that her black-and-white thinking did not help and in fact made her feel worse and more vulnerable and thus reinforced her depression. With the opportunity to grieve some of her losses and practice alternate ways to view her situation, Dorothy was able to acknowledge that some other residents at Oakdale had it worse than she did and that, without making an effort in physical therapy, she was at higher risk of becoming even more frail than she already felt.

The psychologist also worked with Dorothy to think of ways to make the best of her unfortunate, but temporary, nursing home placement. She told Dorothy how much the staff, like any other human beings, liked to be appreciated for the work they did. Using the old saying, "It's easier to catch flies with honey than with vinegar," together they role-played Dorothy giving positive feedback to a nurse after a dressing change. Though she initially felt that she should not have to thank staff for a less than perfect job, Dorothy made modest gains in this skill. As the staff was at the same time making an effort to pay her more positive attention, Dorothy was sometimes able to give them positive feedback.

After the initial month of treatment, Dorothy again completed the GDS and scored 14 of 30 points, indicating decreased depressive thoughts from her earlier baseline (although with continued expression of feeling helpless, worthless, worried, not happy or hopeful). She reported improved appetite and motivation for physical therapy, but continued disrupted sleep and irritability. With these ongoing symptoms, Dorothy agreed to an evaluation with the consulting psychiatrist, who started her on a trial of paroxetine (Paxil). The psychologist continued to meet with her weekly for the next month, during which time she reinforced the gains Dorothy had made as well as supported her tolerating the initial gastrointestinal upset with the Paxil, which resolved after the first week. At the end of that month, Dorothy was discharged home with the assistance of visiting nurse and homemaking services. The psychologist asked that a psychiatric home health nurse also be assigned to monitor her mood, provide support, and communicate concerns to Dorothy's primary care doctor, who would monitor the antidepressant medication.

Comment

Dorothy's depression was helped by a combination of interventions and, while treatment did not attempt to alter her long-standing narcissistic personality, the staff was able to respond to it in a way that minimized disruptions to her care and to the system. Breaking the dysfunctional cycle of communication between Dorothy and her caregivers was key. In such cases, working only with the individual patient is unlikely to be effective. The systemic intervention can ultimately promote change on multiple levels and have the potential to enhance functioning of all participants in the system.

While Dorothy's depressive symptoms did improve, she continued with a generally negative outlook about herself, her situation, and her future. In the context of her personality and long-standing difficulty adapting to changes in her bodily integrity, appearance, and functioning, Dorothy would continue to have great trouble acknowledging any positive aspects of her situation. Personality disorders can indeed complicate the treatment of late-life depression but, especially when interventions can occur on multiple levels, meaningful gains can be made.

CHAPTER FIFTEEN

Posttraumatic Stress Disorder and Depression: Mary Stuart

Many people who survive to old age have been exposed to trauma earlier (or later) in life and can experience new onset, chronic, or exacerbated symptoms of posttraumatic stress disorder (PTSD) in late life. Sometimes late-in-life physical vulnerability or loss can trigger earlier traumatic memories and emotional reactions; sometimes, too, a slowdown in activities can make distraction from such memories and emotions more difficult (Clipp and Elder, 1996; Weintraub and Ruskin, 1999). Depression commonly occurs in the context of PTSD (Ballenger et al., 2000; Stein et al., 2000), and each of these disorders can complicate the treatment of the other (Hyer, 1999). Unfortunately, trauma history and its impact on the older adult's mental health are often not adequately assessed, as was true in Mary's case despite years of psychiatric care. Ultimately, acknowledging her trauma history and addressing PTSD in her treatment plan were important for effective care of her depression.

Mary Stuart: Introduction

Mary, a 68-year-old woman with a history of recurrent major depression, was recently admitted for her sixth psychiatric hospitalization over a period of 48 years. She had become increasingly depressed during the prior year, with poor response to several antidepressant medication trials. When her husband Ralph died two months ago, she became despondent; she was not able to sleep, had stopped eating, and wanted to die. She was also suffering from painful arthritis that limited her mobility.

During the current psychiatric admission, she was treated with electroconvulsive therapy (ECT) because of the risk of her minimal nutritional intake, her poor response to medications, and her positive response to ECT in the past.

While Mary was in the hospital, her three adult children—all of whom lived in the area—came to visit and determined that she would be better off moving to an apartment near her oldest daughter. She agreed, conceding that she had no desire to live in her house without Ralph. Because moving out of her home would compound the adjustment issues Mary was already facing with the loss of her husband, the psychologist who covered the unit was asked to evaluate Mary for psychotherapy.

Issues for Consideration

At this point, we know little more than that Mary has had a long history of recurring major depression that has responded to ECT in the past. Questions we have include: What has typically precipitated her depressive relapses? What is her typical functioning in between episodes of major depression? We would also like to learn more about her medical conditions; her personal, family, work, and psychiatric history; her personal and environmental resources; and her wishes for the future.

Assessment

The inpatient psychiatric assessment focused on Mary's current symptoms of depression, her medical status and mental status, and her thoughts about death and suicide. Prior psychiatric treatment records were available for the team to review. The psychologist read the following:

- First episode of depression at the age of 20, at which point she was hospitalized; details about precipitants, assessment, or treatment were not available.

- Second episode of depression in her late forties, during a brief relapse of her husband's alcohol abuse, when he became disinhibited, demanding, and less dependable. She was hospitalized with suicidal ideation and treated with a tricyclic antidepressant.
- Third episode and hospitalization in her early fifties, following surgery on her knee after falling on the ice. At that time, she felt guilty for being a burden to her husband and children, felt helpless and worthless, and was having disturbed sleep with nightmares. She responded positively to ECT during this hospital stay.
- Fourth episode of depression and hospital stay 10 years ago. At the time, arthritic knee pain was limiting her ability to walk, drive, shop, cook, and clean; she became hopeless, fearful, and was barely eating or sleeping. She was treated successfully with a tricyclic antidepressant. Soon thereafter, she was able to have knee replacement surgery, which helped.
- Fifth episode and hospitalization last year, which did not have an obvious precipitant. She was treated with ECT and discharged on an atypical antidepressant. She maintained contact with her outpatient psychiatrist since then; notes suggested that her depression never fully remitted.
- The present hospitalization was her sixth.

Over the years, Mary had seen various psychiatrists. She was maintained on different antidepressant medications, although not consistently. She and her husband also saw a religious counselor for a few months after his alcohol relapse 20 years ago.

By the time of the interview with the psychologist, Mary had completed half of her 12-treatment ECT series and was already eating again, sleeping better, showing brighter affect, interacting with other patients, and participating in crocheting and painting classes. At the time, she was also being treated with an antibiotic for a urinary tract infection (UTI). She was agreeable to the interview with the psychologist, who explained to Mary that she wanted to ask her questions about her history and current stresses in order to help Mary plan a smooth transition out of the hospital.

Mary shared information about her early history. She was the fifth of seven children in a devout Lutheran family. Her parents were very active in the church in their city neighborhood. Mary was a serious and bright student, and received a scholarship to attend a small women's college several hours from home. She experienced her first episode of depression during her third year at college and, after returning to live with her parents, never returned to school. After working as a clerk at a local drug store, she met and married her husband, and subsequently raised their three children.

In addition to this personal history, the psychologist reviewed Mary's trauma history. She asked Mary, "Did anyone ever touch you in a way that made you feel uncomfortable?" Mary paused, and then responded, "yes." She went on to describe that during college she had a boyfriend who "forced himself" on her multiple times. She ultimately left college and returned home to her parents to get away. It was at that time that she had her first psychiatric inpatient treatment for depression. She voiced that she had attempted to "blank it out of her mind," that she "knew it was wrong," had "no one to tell," and had "nowhere to go but back home." Mary said that no one had asked her of this before, and she had always been too ashamed to mention it. She denied a history of physical, sexual, or emotional abuse as a younger child, although did report that her parents were very strict.

On the basis of this initial psychological assessment, the psychologist thought that, in addition to her severe, recurrent major depression, Mary might suffer from PTSD secondary to the rape trauma, but this would need further assessment. The psychologist also wondered whether Mary's UTI—and a possible delirium—had contributed to the severe presentation of her depression at the time of admission. Finally, she wanted to learn more about Mary's marital relationship, her grief response, and feelings about moving from her home to an apartment near her daughter.

Conceptualization

At this point in Mary's care, the relationship between her trauma history and recurrent major depression is not yet clear, but important to consider. Over many years of psychiatric treatment, she either had not been asked or had not felt comfortable to share information about her rape history. It is possible that depressive episodes were triggered by trauma-related stress, for example, during times when she was relatively vulnerable or immobilized (knee surgery, arthritis) and when her husband was relatively more threatening to her (due to personality change when he was drinking).

Although identifying the trauma likely would have important implications for understanding Mary's style of coping and relating over her lifetime, it may or may not have immediate treatment implications. Given the multiple issues facing Mary during this acute hospital stay—medical stabilization, her ability to eat and sleep, her acute grief, her suicidal feelings, her residential decisions—the first priority was to help assure her safety and ability to regain self-care capacities.

Communication and trust were also important issues for Mary's care. She had a long history of treatment with psychiatric providers, but no history of psychotherapy treatment. She was, however, quite open to discussing her concerns. She would need some brief education to help socialize her into the role of an active participant in psychotherapy.

Treatment

Mary agreed to meet with the psychologist as she made the transition from inpatient to partial hospital to outpatient treatment. She was fortunate to be in a system in which the psychologist could work across multiple settings, facilitating continuity of care. Initially, the treatment goals focused on stabilization, adjustment to her new residence, and grief. Mary believed moving was a good decision, was adjusting to living on her own without Ralph, and was coping well with resolving grief. Mary continued to use skills she had learned in the hospital, including monitoring her mood on a daily basis and working to identify and increase activities she had found enjoyable in the past but had discontinued (e.g., word puzzles, needlework, cleaning and decorating her apartment). Further, as her ECT treatment was discontinued, she started taking an antidepressant medication.

The outpatient psychotherapy began to help Mary identify core beliefs that contributed to her depressive outlook, including themes of being a victim, out of control, helpless, and vulnerable. The therapist gradually asked Mary more about these beliefs and questioned if they developed before or after her rape experiences. As Mary's depression remitted, treatment was able to shift to PTSD issues.

While Mary responded to the therapist's questioning about her rape experience with anxiety and an avoidant coping style that may have originated or been exacerbated in response to her trauma ("I try not to think about those things"), she did agree to further assessment of possible PTSD. During one treatment session, the psychologist administered a structured clinical interview for PTSD (Clinician-Administered PTSD Scale-CAPS; Blake et al., 1995), which found Mary to meet criteria for PTSD due to her rape trauma. She was currently endorsing:

- intense psychological distress when reading newspaper articles about people who had been raped (reexperiencing);
- persistent avoidant thinking of her rape experiences, moderate feelings of detachment/estrangement from others, a restricted range of affect, and the sense of foreshortened future much of the time (avoidance/numbing);
- insomnia, difficulty concentrating, hypervigilance, and an exaggerated startle response (hyperarousal).

For Mary, the assessment itself was difficult but also therapeutic because she learned that, in fact, her symptom pattern did meet diagnostic criteria for PTSD; this "label" helped to validate the difficult experiences she had had since her rape. Mary and the therapist discussed the interplay of her PTSD and her depression. For example, when Mary would run across a rape article in the paper, her hypervigilance and numbing would increase, leading to aggravated sleep disturbance, difficulty concentrating, and emotional distancing from people, all of which could exacerbate or contribute to her depression. This helped Mary understand that, in order for her condition to become more stable, it might help her to address her PTSD experience. However, Mary didn't believe that treatment could help her with problems she'd had for over 40 years. At the same time, she had developed a strong therapeutic alliance with the therapist and believed the therapist wanted to help her.

Using Cognitive Processing Therapy (CPT) for rape victims (Resick and Schnicke, 1993) as a model for treatment, the therapist worked with Mary to process the affect of her trauma in a structured way while challenging the beliefs she held about herself and her experience. The goal of the treatment is to help patients accommodate, in a cognitive and emotional sense, their traumatic experience, that is, to understand and experience that bad things sometimes happen to people who are good or nondeserving of terrible experiences.

Mary's reaction to her rape experience needed to be understood in her generational context. At the time she went to college, there was no awareness or discussion of the phenomenon of "date rape." Mary very much believed that she must have done something to deserve the assaults and maintained a sense of self-blame, distrust, fear, and avoidance throughout her adulthood. Her strict religious upbringing further engrained her sense of responsibility and guilt. When the issue and language of "date rape" started to receive attention in the 1980s, Mary followed the news coverage and commentary closely, trying to make sense of her experience in spite of the reexperiencing and hypervigilance it created in her. The therapy provided a structured and safe setting for Mary to challenge her beliefs about safety, trust, power, esteem, and intimacy.

One year after her hospital stay, Mary had made much improvement; her remaining symptoms of PTSD and depression were mild, and she had developed strategies to cope with them. She continued on her antidepressant medication and in maintenance psychotherapy for depression and PTSD, initially biweekly, then tapered to monthly, bimonthly, and quarterly. She has had no recurrence of major depression for six years. She currently has plans to discontinue psychotherapy at some point ("I don't plan to be in therapy for the rest of my life") and, at the same time, finds that booster sessions three times per year help to reinforce her continued well-being.

Comment

Trauma assessment in older adults with depression is important. Though Mary might have had recurrent major depression without her trauma history–and, certainly, not all people with trauma develop severe depression–she was able to benefit from treatment for PTSD late in her life. In our clinical experience, when older adult patients with PTSD receive education about the symptoms and impact of the disorder, they often make comments along the lines of: "I would have been a different person, and been able to live a different life, if I had been able to have treatment for this horrible experience earlier in my life."

However, it may not always be appropriate to do trauma work with older adults with long-standing PTSD. Because PTSD treatment is stressful and symptoms do emerge during treatment, individuals must be psychiatrically stable, without suicidal ideation, and have solid support structures in addition to the therapist. Further, long-standing patterns of coping with PTSD symptoms may serve some older adults quite well; in such cases, it may not be helpful to "rock the boat." As always, sound clinical judgment, consultation, and discretion are essential in these situations.

CHAPTER SIXTEEN

Bipolar Disorder: Elaine Conway

Older adults can experience depression or mania that is part of a long-standing bipolar disorder. Such a history of affective disorder can take many forms, with combinations of prior episodes of major depression, mania, hypomania, and/or subsyndromal depression, and with varying baseline levels of functioning. Elaine's case illustrates the first manic episode in a 75-year-old woman who had a history of depression and hypomania. Triggered in part by worries for her husband's health, her experience demonstrates how long-standing patterns of coping—at either an individual or couple/family level—may be less adaptive during times of stress in late life. Family psychoeducation and couple's therapy were important interventions, in addition to hospitalization and treatment with a mood-stabilizing medication.

Elaine Conway: Introduction

Elaine, a 75-year-old European-American woman, had obtained a master's degree in English literature at Smith College. She and her husband, John, had had an extremely close marriage for the past 53 years, and Elaine enjoyed the role of wife and mother. They welcomed John's retirement 10 years ago, and had purchased a condo in Florida for winters away from their home in Albany, New York.

They both enjoyed excellent physical health until five years ago, when John fell from the roof and suffered multiple fractures to his leg. Weeks later, he fell again and broke a hip. The surgery for the hip repair went well, yet was very taxing for Elaine. She was exhausted; overnight, she had become a full-time caregiver and was fearful of losing her beloved husband. She worked almost constantly to help him and to maintain their home. Thankfully, John responded well to rehabilitation and, within a year, was again walking, although with somewhat less gusto than before. As John grew stronger, Elaine felt more secure and was better able to relax.

Elaine sometimes worried about her ability to handle stress, knowing she had a positive family history for manic depression: Her mother and a brother had been on lithium. Elaine had had two episodes of postpartum depression, after her third and fourth children's births. Throughout her adult life, she had brief periods of hypomania, with increased energy, racing thoughts, and a moderately expansive mood. During these times, her family and friends described her as the "life of the party" and enjoyed her gregarious and exuberant nature, but also found her exhausting. She had never been on any psychotropic medication.

Last summer, Elaine and John decided to enjoy time traveling. Despite minor health concerns—Elaine's arthritis and John's hypertension—they were both feeling relatively well and they wanted to explore a new city. They purchased a time-share and decided to visit Montreal, Canada, for a month. At the beginning of their stay, John had his first episode of congestive heart failure (CHF). Although she was able to obtain good care for him in Canada, it was stressful negotiating the health system away from home.

Elaine became increasingly frightened about John's health and worried about making it home should he have another difficult episode on the road. She frequently stayed up at night, watching him breathe and worrying about him. At the same time, John was concerned about Elaine, who was becoming more irritable, sleeping only two to three hours per night, and talking a blue streak; their time-share neighbors seemed to give each other strange looks when she was around. He figured she was having a hard time away from home and thought they should plan an early return. When one night he found her walking naked around the pool area, he was terrified. He called his eldest daughter, Anne, in Washington, D.C., and her husband flew up to Canada the next day to drive them home. Elaine was admitted to the psychiatric inpatient unit for her first manic episode.

After one week in the hospital, she began to respond positively to lithium, was participating in classes on the unit, and had met regularly with her case manager. Anne flew in from D.C. for the weekend, and approached the case manager with her concern not only about her mom, but also about her dad. Anne said that she and her three sisters frequently had conversations with each of their parents, in which one was worrying about the other. However, she was pretty sure her mom and dad never talked to each other about their respective worries. Anne thought they were both under an enormous amount of stress. The case manager referred Elaine and John for couple's therapy, and an appointment with the psychologist covering the unit was scheduled for the following day.

Issues for Consideration

Multiple stressors led to Elaine and John's current situation. What were possible triggers for Elaine's manic episode? How does Elaine cope when John becomes injured or ill? How do John and Elaine typically cope with relational stressors, and how do they usually communicate with each other? What is the nature of Elaine and John's extended social support system? The onset of mania (or major depression) and subsequent hospitalization of a loved one are significant stressors for a family. Elaine's entire family could benefit from education regarding what to expect from the hospitalization, how to understand Elaine's illness, and how to manage her illness after discharge.

Assessment

At the onset of the initial interview with the couple, the psychologist attempted to establish rapport with both Elaine and John, and to normalize the feelings they might have about the hospitalization experience. She wanted to hear each of their perspectives, as well as to observe how they interacted. She acknowledged that hospitalization is a stressful time, and that it was not uncommon for both husband and wife, as well as adult children, to need some time to sort out and understand the experience: Why had it happened? How had it happened? What does this mean for the couple, and for the family? What can be done to prevent it in the future?

The psychologist observed that Elaine was hyperverbal and anxious (e.g., her posture was tense), yet was fairly well-groomed. John walked with a slight limp, was well dressed, and grimaced slightly when Elaine interrupted him or the psychologist. The couple appeared to genuinely care about each other, sitting close on the couch and frequently touching each other's hand, arm, or shoulder. They shared in answering questions about their history.

They met on a blind date set up by mutual friends and, with fairly immediate attraction to each other, began dating and were married within the year. They both had fond memories of their courtship and engagement period. After marrying, the couple settled and raised their four daughters in Washington, D.C., John's hometown.

John's parents had helped to care for the young children during Elaine's two episodes of postpartum depression. Each time, Elaine spent several months frequently crying and in bed, but eventually got better without treatment. She never again experienced that degree of depression.

John and Elaine described themselves as inseparable: They enjoyed golfing, current events, politics, and good fiction and historical nonfiction. They had maintained fairly stereotypic gender roles throughout their marriage. Elaine described John as her "protector." John voiced pride in being the "man of the house" and described Elaine as his "beloved" and his "dear one." Their plan had always been to return to Elaine's hometown near Albany, where she had extended family and wanted to be near her aging parents. Once their daughters were out of the house, John secured an offer with a good firm in Albany, and they moved. They had now lived for just over 20 years in a beautiful rural area not far from the city.

They spoke of close relationships with their four daughters, each of whom they viewed as competent, intelligent, and solid citizens. Three of the four remained in the D.C. area, and one had stayed in Denver after graduate school. Despite the distance, Elaine and John relied on them and their husbands increasingly for emotional support, with frequent phone calls, letters, and visits.

Finally, they described the health changes that had affected them over the past five years, starting with John's accident. The therapist noted that they were perceptive and protective of the other's experience of illness. For example, Elaine noted that John really hated being hospitalized for his hip surgery and rehab because he missed his routine at home and despised feeling so weak. Even during that time, she knew he was trying to "act strong" for her and the family. John stated that he didn't think he would ever tell Elaine about all that had happened when she was manic. During the session, John also admitted that Elaine's history of occasional euphoric mood, irritability, loud talking, and interrupting others was frightening to him in social situations; he felt helpless when he couldn't seem to quiet her down. And, in spite of Elaine's strong family history of bipolar disorder, they admitted knowing little about the illness itself.

At the end of the first meeting, the psychologist raised the possibility of including as many of their daughters as possible in the next session, either in person or on a conference call, because they were such strong supports. Elaine and John agreed, and they arranged to meet again with the therapist to discuss the recent stresses they were facing.

Conceptualization

Elaine's genetic vulnerability, combined with John's physical health problems that stressed Elaine and deprived her of sleep, likely contributed to her manic episode. From Elaine's perspective, seeing her "protector" as frail and vulnerable was frightening. Becoming the caregiver in the relationship, and facing her fears of losing him, had overwhelmed her usual coping resources. From John's perspective, it was frightening and embarrassing to watch his intelligent and socially skilled wife become so mentally ill, that is, making no sense and being totally inappropriate in social situations.

The couple's long-standing interdependence and mutual protectiveness likely contributed to difficult adjustment when faced with these illnesses and fears of loss. Their ability to be sensitive to the other's needs and feelings, and to want to avoid upsetting the other, was appreciated by each of them. But we might also wonder—as did their daughters—how stressful it must be not to talk to one's spouse about certain stresses and fears.

Related to the importance of straightforward communication, Elaine and her family would need to understand the mental illness. Therefore, initial therapy treatment goals would include: providing the family with education about bipolar and affective disorders and their treatment (Hinrichsen and Zweig, 1994); continuing to stabilize Elaine's mood (monitoring her response to the medication in collaboration with the treating psychiatrist); and helping Elaine and John to develop skills for communicating more directly with each other, as tools for coping with future times of stress.

Treatment

The next week the psychologist learned from the case manager that Elaine would transfer to the partial-hospitalization program by midweek, and that she and John appeared to be accepting of this. Elaine was responding well to the lithium, with increased control over her speech and affect, and improved insight and judgment regarding her behavior.

During the couple's next session with the psychologist, daughters Anne and Elizabeth attended in person, while Joanne and Peggy participated via conference call. The psychologist introduced this family meeting as a time to share information about the hospitalization process, bipolar illness, and discharge plans and recommendations; to ask questions they might have; and to provide input regarding the situation. During the discussion, the psychologist observed positive interactions among the family members: They were respectful of and seemed to enjoy each other. Elaine's speech was less pressured and intrusive than the previous week, and everyone expressed relief at seeing mom getting "back to her usual self." The psychologist spent time reviewing the importance of follow-up care and how the family could recognize signs of relapse. Everyone agreed that Elaine and John would benefit from continued couple's sessions for a brief period of time.

Elaine attended the partial-hospital program three days a week for one month, during which time she and John met weekly for couple's therapy; the couple's work then continued twice monthly for three additional months. In addition to practicing active listening skills, the psychologist worked with the couple to understand both the benefits and risks of the protectiveness they had toward each other. It was very helpful in some very concrete ways, for example, when Elaine removed throw rugs at home so John wouldn't trip after his injuries, or when John offered to cook when Elaine's arthritis was particularly painful. However, the protectiveness was also hurtful, for example, when John resisted telling Elaine when she started exhibiting signs of mania, not wanting to embarrass her. Or, when Elaine resisted telling John how scared she was to lose him when he was sick.

They admitted that keeping such concerns private felt isolating and burdensome, but that they had difficulty being more direct with each other. In sessions, they practiced expressing their needs and concerns more directly, initially experienced as a foreign task. With time and encouragement from the therapist and each other, both were able to develop skill and comfort with more direct communication. They realized it helped them to feel even closer and to plan more openly for the future. For example, given Elaine's fears of losing John, they talked with the family about options for Elaine should John die before her. Though this was difficult, it did help Elaine to realize she had many supports and would never be completely alone.

Comment

Illness or disability in one member of an older couple can easily shake up the usual roles, expectations, and habits in the relationship. Most couples are able to adapt to changes in their respective abilities, and subsequent impact on their relationship, without significant difficulty. However, rigid role expectations or rigid communication styles can make such adaptation more difficult (Qualls, 1995; Rosowsky, 1999). And, of course, an individual with a family history of psychiatric illness, like Elaine, may be vulnerable to relapse when faced with certain threats or when her usual coping strategies are no longer helpful.

The types of stresses that precipitated Elaine's mania are likely to become worse, rather than better, as the couple faces continued chronic health problems and related disability. Predicting such stresses, anticipating ways of coping with them, and educating families about risk of and signs of relapse are all important for managing serious affective disorder in late life. This couple was fortunate to have many resources at their disposal, including intelligence, financial stability, a supportive family, and capacity for insight.

Chapter Seventeen

Psychotic Depression: Joanna Tysen

Severe depression can occur with psychotic features. In older adults, psychotic depression often entails delusions related to somatic concerns or fears of persecution (Meyers and Greenberg, 1986). Such experiences can be quite frightening to patients and family members alike. And, delusional thinking contributes to poor insight about the impact of depressive illness on one's thoughts, feelings, and behaviors. Late-life psychotic depression appears to have greater risk for relapse or recurrence than nonpsychotic depression (Flint and Rifat, 1998b). Though evidence suggests that ECT or antidepressant plus antipsychotic medication are efficacious for the initial treatment of psychotic depression in late life (Flint and Rifat, 1998a), preventing relapse can remain a clinical challenge. In some cases, individuals treated for psychotic depression sustain poor insight after treatment; unaware of how sick they were, they dismiss the importance of continuing maintenance therapy. Joanna's case illustrates how an older woman with psychotic depression, who had stopped eating and drinking, ultimately had to be hospitalized against her will and treated with ECT. Intensive psychotherapeutic and psychopharmacological follow-up helped to prevent another relapse.

Joanna Tysen: Introduction

Joanna, an 84-year-old married Irish-Catholic woman, was a retired nurse manager with three grown sons. Her first treated episode of major depression followed the deaths about 10 years ago of two aunts for whom she had been helping to care; a tricyclic antidepressant medication helped her to recover at that time. Five months ago, she was hospitalized to treat a severe recurrence of the depression that did not respond to the previous antidepressant medication. She had become increasingly preoccupied with and distressed by vague concerns about her throat and eating habits, limiting the foods she would attempt to eat. Precipitants to the depressive episode included a wrist fracture sustained in a fall from a ladder and the recent death of a close friend. She responded to an SSRI medication trial with the additional support and structure of an inpatient and then partial-hospitalization program for six weeks.

Soon after discharge from the program, however, Joanna discontinued her medication and stopped attending her regular aftercare psychotherapy because she was feeling better. Over several months, she again became increasingly depressed—she ate less and less, then drank less and less, and then started to complain that she could not swallow because she had no throat.

Her husband Fred was concerned about her weight loss and irrational thinking and behavior. While previously he could encourage her to eat and drink, she now refused almost all nutrition. She was also refusing to see her psychiatrist. With the help of one of their sons, he dressed her and, despite her protests, took her to the hospital, where she refused to be admitted. Given the life-threatening nature of her depression, however, Fred petitioned for her involuntary admission, and both a psychiatrist and an internist certified to the court that she was gravely disabled and a danger to herself, and that her treatment was necessary.

Issues for Consideration

Depression is a chronic illness, and the risk of relapse is high (one episode: 50% risk of relapse; two episodes: 70% risk of relapse; three or more episodes: 90% risk of relapse).

The first 6–12 months following recovery from an episode of major depression are typically the highest risk period for relapse. Therefore, it is common for treatments to be continued up to a year or more after initial remission of the episode. This is particularly true for a second or third episode, as in Joanna's case. Joanna lacked insight into her risk for relapse, and discontinued her treatment. How might she have been helped to continue her medication and psychotherapy?

Moreover: What was the meaning of the losses of Joanna's aunts and her friend? What was most difficult about her disabling wrist injury? What is the nature of her relationship with her husband and her sons? What education or support might her family need to understand and supervise her care? When Joanna was well, how was she spending her time in retirement and what were her typical strategies for coping with stress and loss?

Assessment

When Joanna came to the hospital for an evaluation, she and Fred met with the psychiatrist who knew them from her previous admission. After briefly reviewing Joanna's old chart, the psychiatrist recalled that Joanna did have a positive response to the SSRI tried during the prior admission. The chart indicated a family history significant for depressive illness in her father and one of her sons. Additionally, although she had not been treated, she and her husband had recalled a period of depression after the birth of her third son.

The chart also detailed precipitants to the prior admission: Almost two years ago, one of her closest friends had died from cancer, following recurrent episodes of lymphoma during which Joanna had provided nursing care. Then, last winter, she slipped on a ladder while cleaning and broke her wrist. The fracture was painful and, for several months, interfered with her ability to drive and do usual household tasks. The injury contributed to inactivity, difficulty helping others in her usual way, and, ultimately, a sense of uselessness, helplessness, decreased interest, and depressed mood.

Joanna did return to see her psychiatrist during that time, encouraged by her primary care doctor to do so. However, she did not respond to the tricyclic antidepressant that had helped her before, nor to an initial trial of an SSRI. Meanwhile, she spent excessive time in bed and developed a passive death wish. She willingly accepted her psychiatrist's offer of admission to the hospital, where the structure and treatment of the therapeutic milieu, coupled with another medication trial, seemed to help her: The treatment team "required" her, like all the other patients, to get out of bed, to begin a moderate exercise program, and to participate in structured skills-building classes that continued into the partial-hospital program. After six weeks, she was brighter, less depressed, more energetic, and more motivated to pursue previously enjoyable activities. She was happy to be discharged from the program and spend more time doing spring cleaning at home.

That was six months ago. On interview now, Joanna looked tired, disheveled, pale, and underweight. With her 30-pound weight loss, her clothes literally hung on her. When the psychiatrist asked her what had happened in the past six months, Joanna responded briefly that she didn't know. She voiced frustration that Fred kept pushing her to eat and to drink, and that this was impossible because she "couldn't swallow" and she "had no throat." The psychiatrist got her a glass of water; Joanna took a small sip, swallowed, and said, "See what I mean? I can't swallow. I don't have a throat. I just don't know what happened to it—it's gone." Fred looked exhausted and exasperated, and said this had also been her response at home.

Fred asserted that, after Joanna's discharge, he became concerned when she began to spend more time in bed, leaving her closet-cleaning and photograph-organizing projects unfinished. He was used to depending on her to cook the meals, keep in touch with the children and grandchildren, and generally take care of him and the home. He now had to do more of these things on his own. He did not realize until recently that she had stopped taking her medication and quit attending her therapy meetings. Usually, she was very responsible about her health and her commitments. He became worried as she ate less and less and, just recently, could not be convinced to eat or drink. Afraid he might lose her, he and his son brought her to the hospital.

On the basis of the interview, the psychiatrist agreed that an inpatient admission was needed. He was concerned about Joanna's life-threatening situation: her weight loss, her decreased food and fluid intake, and her delusional thinking. He considered a diagnosis of psychotic depression, delirium, some other acute medical problem, or a combination of the above. A medical evaluation showed no acute medical problem except that she would likely soon require intravenous rehydration if she continued to refuse fluids. With this medical clearance, she was admitted, as described above, to the psychiatric inpatient unit against her will.

Conceptualization

Joanna's status required immediate medical evaluation, given both her compromised nutritional status and the fact that acute psychotic symptoms can sometimes indicate a delirium secondary to a medical condition or medication. With no evidence of the latter, and considering her increased depression and her somatic preoccupation during her prior admission, her probable diagnosis was recurrent major depression, severe, with psychotic features. Her history did indicate a biological vulnerability to depressive illness.

The brief social history obtained suggested that Joanna was typically the caregiver to her family and friends, as well as in her professional life as a nurse. Her depressive episodes appeared to be precipitated by losses of people who had been under her care and/or by her inability to remain active and responsible for others (i.e., when she broke her wrist). Her husband tended to depend on her to care for him (a long-standing pattern), and had initial difficulty accepting her deterioration and the need for him to take charge of the situation (e.g., by seeing if she was taking her medicines). It is not clear if her outpatient psychiatrist and social worker therapist had tried to follow up with her when she did not come in. It is easy for such patients to "fall through the cracks," sometimes with devastating consequences.

These psychological and systemic issues would need to be addressed once the current crisis was resolved. As Joanna was severely disabled, without adequate insight or judgment, she had to be hospitalized against her will.

Treatment

Once admitted to the inpatient geropsychiatric unit, Joanna was hostile toward others, mistrustful, isolating in her room, and severely depressed. Given her delusional symptoms and her refusal to eat, the psychiatrist felt that ECT was indicated; trying another medication that could take weeks or more to work seemed too risky. As required by state law, a second psychiatric evaluation was completed, which concurred with the initial impression and treatment plan.

Joanna, Fred, and two of their sons met with a nurse who educated them about ECT. Together, they watched a short video that outlined the possible benefits and risks involved with the treatment, and while Joanna had a difficult time accepting that she was someone who needed such treatment, her husband and sons encouraged her to give it a chance. Able to understand the risks and benefits of the treatment, she signed a consent form.

Joanna began a course of ECT three times a week. After the first week, her family reported that she looked brighter and she was less hostile to hospital staff. She did report having a headache after initial treatments (helped with Tylenol), and family and staff noted that she had some trouble remembering events just before and afterward, but otherwise her mental status appeared to be improving. She was consuming more fluids and voicing less frequent delusional beliefs about her throat. During the second week of ECT, she began to feel less agitated and mistrustful, to eat without prompting, and to participate in structured classes with other patients in which she occasionally smiled and engaged socially. With positive response after eight treatments, the team decided to discontinue her ECT and begin her antidepressant medication once again.

Once Joanna was discharged, a visiting nurse came weekly for the first month to ensure that she was taking her medication. The responsibility was then transferred collaboratively to Fred and Joanna. Fred accompanied her to the clinic for her weekly outpatient psychotherapy appointments with the social worker; occasionally he joined these sessions to give his impressions of her progress, as well as to discuss some couple's issues that arose. Joanna was able to speak about her identity as a caregiver, and how difficult it was for her to feel powerless over the loss of her family members and friends. She was helped to grieve these losses, as well as to evaluate her unrealistic expectations of "being perfect." Fred and she spoke of their long-standing dynamic in which she was more in charge, and how they were trying to adjust this for both their benefits.

Joanna was helped to understand that she was at risk for relapse of depression and that, to adequately care for her family, she needed to make the commitment to care for her depressive illness. Fred and Joanna were encouraged to be alert for signs of relapse (for Joanna, increased isolation and time in bed, decreased appetite, and complaints about her throat). After four months, her therapy appointments were tapered to biweekly, then monthly, then bimonthly. She was doing quite well with the antidepressant medication, semiannual appointments with the psychiatrist, and bimonthly appointments with the social worker. Four years after this treatment, she remained stable with no further recurrence of life-threatening depression.

Comment

When severe depression is life-threatening and/or has failed multiple medication or psychotherapy trials, ECT is an indicated treatment. ECT has been shown to be safe and effective for depressed elders, including those with comorbid neurological problems or cerebrovascular disease (Kelly and Zisselman, 2000). Contraindications for ECT include unstable cardiovascular conditions, conditions causing increased intracranial pressure, recent cerebral hemorrhage or infarction, severe pulmonary condition, and high anesthetic risk (Kelly and Zisselman, 2000). ECT is known to cause memory loss around the time of the treatments, but there do not appear to be enduring memory deficits; more research is needed, however. Older adults, especially those with dementia, are at increased risk for delirium after ECT treatments and must be carefully monitored. Although maintenance ECT may be indicated in some patients with recurring severe depressive episodes that do not respond to medication, there is little research to date regarding its long-term effectiveness or risks. In this case, had intervention occurred before there was a crisis, ECT may not have been necessary.

Joanna's severe depression relapsed when she discontinued maintenance medication and psychotherapy and her depression became psychotic and life-threatening in the absence of timely intervention. Once the situation was under control, intensive follow-up and support, combined with a positive response to antidepressant medication, enabled Joanna to stay well. Engaging available family or other support networks to provide monitoring and early identification of signs of relapse, and building careful follow-up into the treatment plan, can contribute significantly to successful management of severe, recurrent depression.

Appendix A: Antidepressant Medications

Depressed older adults can benefit from antidepressant medication, alone or in combination with psychotherapeutic interventions. In this appendix, we review guidelines for considering antidepressant treatment with the older adult, as well as information about the use of specific medications.

Background

Risk of Inappropriate Psychotropic Medication Use by Older Adults

Until recently, the psychotropic medications most commonly prescribed for older adults were sedative hypnotics or anxiolytics, such as diazepam (Valium), chlordiazepam (Librium), lorazepam (Ativan), or temazepam (Restoril). Although these drugs can be effective for certain symptoms of depression (e.g., insomnia or anxiety), they do not treat the underlying depression and, in fact, may worsen or perpetuate depressive symptoms. These drugs can have serious side effects in older adults, including daytime sedation, cognitive impairment and confusion, impaired coordination leading to accidents or falls, and physical or psychological dependence. For these reasons, *the long-term use of sedative hypnotics and benzodiazepines to treat depression should be avoided whenever possible, and antidepressant medications should be used instead.*

Antidepressant Medications

Over 20 antidepressant medications have been shown to be effective in the treatment of depression. The best evidence for the efficacy of antidepressants exists for major depression and dysthymia, but these medications can also be efficacious for minor depression or depression in the face of dementia. Some antidepressants are effective for depression with comorbid anxiety disorders or for primary anxiety disorders (panic disorder, posttraumatic stress disorder, generalized anxiety disorder, and obsessive compulsive disorder).

Antidepressants can be grouped into several classes: tricyclic antidepressants (TCAs), other heterocyclic antidepressants, monoamine oxidase inhibitors (MAOIs), selective serotonin reuptake inhibitors (SSRIs), and other newer antidepressants. Even though most of the research has been done with younger patients, these medications are also effective in older adults (Lebowitz et al., 1997; Reynolds and Lebowitz, 1999; Salzman, 1997). If used at an appropriate dose for a period of 8–12 weeks, antidepressants can lead to substantial improvements in depressive symptoms in 50–70% of patients with major depression. Antidepressant medications, usually prescribed by a primary care provider or psychiatrist, are generally well tolerated and do not cause physical dependence.

Antidepressants and Psychotherapy

Both antidepressant medications and certain types of psychotherapy are effective treatments for late-life depression; depression with psychotic symptoms is the only condition in which antidepressants have a clear advantage over psychotherapy. In most cases, the choice of intervention is influenced by the patient's prior treatment history, preferences, and the local availability of treatment resources.

Sometimes patients start on a course of psychotherapy, show some improvement in depression, but continue to have significant symptoms (e.g., anhedonia, sleep or appetite disturbance, poor concentration, decreased energy). In these cases, it can help to add an antidepressant medication. Alternatively, patients may have a good response to an antidepressant medication but are struggling with significant life stressors or continued functional impairment and can benefit from the addition of a course of psychotherapy. Sometimes, a combination of medications and psychotherapy can be more effective than either treatment alone (e.g., in chronic severe depression), or if a patient prefers to start both treatments at the same time. Combining these treatments requires effective communication and collaboration between the prescribing physician and the psychotherapist. When thus collaborating, it is helpful for both professionals to educate the patient about biological and psychological contributions to depression, and that antidepressants and psychotherapy have complementary roles in the treatment.

General Guidelines for the Effective Use of Antidepressant Medications

One of the biggest challenges for using antidepressants is to ensure that the patient receives an adequate trial of the medication. Patients frequently discontinue antidepressants too early (e.g., during the first month of treatment) or never reach a therapeutic dose. Patients may stop the medication for reasons including ambivalence about taking it, concern about side effects, discouragement if depression does not improve rapidly, or improvement in symptoms and believing that the medication is no longer needed. It is very important during the early weeks and months of treatment to work closely with older adults to ensure they are tolerating and taking the antidepressant medication as prescribed.

A number of strategies can help with adherence to medications at this stage:

- *Communicate respect and caring.* The physician should not *just* write a prescription, but encourage patients and significant others to express concerns and ask questions. This openness will communicate that the physician cares and can be trusted to understand the patient.
- *Educate patients and significant others about antidepressants.* Education, which can be provided by the prescribing physician or by a care manager who works closely with the physician, should address the common concerns of older adults, such as stigma, price, worries about addiction, and the risk of drug–drug interactions when taking multiple medications. A number of educational materials are available in print and videotape format (see organizational resources in Appendix D).
- *Explore and anticipate specific barriers* to medication adherence. Assess whether patients may have problems with cognition (i.e., deficits in memory or executive functioning), vision, fine motor skill, or strength (e.g., unable to open bottles, or pills dropping to the floor), overly complex medication regimens, or ability to pay for the medicine. If any such barriers exist, it is helpful to solicit outside support (e.g., get permission to contact a son or daughter to help organize a pill box).
- *Provide close follow-up* during the early weeks of treatment. Patients on antidepressants should have at least biweekly follow-up during the initial stage of treatment and monthly contacts thereafter. Follow-up contacts can be by the prescribing physician, or by a therapist or caseworker in close communication with the prescribing physician;

they ideally occur in person, but the telephone can also be used effectively for this purpose. During follow-ups, providers should assess the presence of depressive symptoms (ideally using a structured instrument such as a DSM-IV symptom checklist or a brief depression rating scale–see Appendix B) and ask about side effects or other concerns about the medications. Patients who experience significant side effects, or who do not respond adequately to the medication, should be reevaluated by the prescribing physician or a consulting psychiatrist. Follow-up should be proactive (i.e., the clinician should schedule and initiate the call or visit because many depressed elders are not sufficiently motivated, assertive, or organized to initiate such).

General guidelines for the effective use of antidepressants include the following:

- Start the medication at a low dose and build up to an effective dose (see Tables A.1–A.3) over a period of 1–3 weeks.
- Closely monitor adherence and side effects during the initial 6–12 weeks of treatment. Make changes in treatment if needed.
- Patients should show clear signs of improvement after 6–12 weeks on the medication. If they do not, carefully reevaluate the patient for causes of antidepressant nonresponse (see Table A.5) and consider a change in treatment.
- Continue the medication at full dose for at least 6–9 months after resolution of depressive symptoms.
- Patients who are at high risk for relapse (those with more than two prior episodes of depression, dysthymia, and/or residual depressive symptoms) should stay on maintenance antidepressant medication for at least 2 years. Some older adults with chronic or frequently recurring depression may need lifelong antidepressant therapy.

Special considerations for the use of antidepressants in older adults include the following:

- Older adults often take a number of other prescription or nonprescription medications, putting them at increased risk for drug–drug interactions or for poor medication adherence. Carefully review the patient's entire medication regimen when prescribing any new drug.

- Older adults, particularly those with impaired kidney or liver function, may have decreased metabolism of antidepressants, leading to slower elimination and increased blood levels of medications. This can be a particular problem with tricyclic antidepressants, which can be dangerous at high blood levels. In general, starting and final doses of antidepressants are somewhat lower in older than in younger adults (see Tables A.1–A.3).
- Older adults may be more sensitive to side effects, particularly with tricyclic antidepressants (see description below). Carefully monitor older adults for such side effects and adjust treatment as needed (see Table A.4).

Choosing an Antidepressant

The available antidepressant medications differ in their cost, side effect profiles, safety in overdose, and drug–drug interactions. Some of the newer medications (see Tables A.2 and A.3), protected by patent laws and not yet available in generic form, are more expensive; expense is a common barrier for older adults without medication insurance coverage. Because all antidepressant medications are roughly equally efficacious in clinical research studies, the choice of a specific antidepressant should be based on a number of factors:

- specific symptoms of depression (e.g., select an activating antidepressant in patients with psychomotor retardation or hypersomnia);
- patient preference;
- prior treatment experience in patients or close family members (prior response to a particular medication may be a good predictor of success);
- anticipated side effects and drug–drug interactions;
- cost and availability of medications.

When cost concerns are not a major barrier, SSRIs or other newer antidepressants are usually recommended as first-line agents for patients with major depression because of their relative safety and tolerability. The following section provides information about specific types of antidepressants.

Tricyclic Antidepressants (TCAs)

TCAs have been used to treat depression for many years (see Table A.1) and have been shown to be efficacious in 50–70% of patients with major depression. They are usually taken once daily in the evening because of their sedating side effects. The disadvantages of TCAs are common side effects, including arrhythmias (particularly in patients with preexisting cardiac conduction defects), dry mouth, constipation, blurred vision, orthostatic hypotension, and weight gain. Other side effects can include sedation, weakness, fatigue, tachycardia, and agitation.

Whenever possible, secondary amine tricyclics such as nortriptyline or desipramine (listed in bold in Table A.1) are preferable to other tricyclics because they have relatively fewer side effects. This is particularly important for older individuals, who are both more sensitive to TCA side effects and more likely to be taking other medications with TCA-like side effects.

Because all TCAs can affect cardiac conduction, they should be avoided in patients with a recent history of myocardial infarction or with preexisting cardiac conduction defects. Patients should have their cardiac conduction evaluated with an electrocardiogram before and after starting a TCA and should be monitored for the emergence of orthostatic hypotension. Because of their anticholinergic side effects, TCAs are also contraindicated in patients who suffer from narrow angle glaucoma or urinary retention. Finally, tricyclics are **extremely dangerous in case of an overdose.** Ten days worth of a TCA may constitute a fatal overdose.

Serum levels of TCAs can be useful if patients don't have a response at a "therapeutic" dose or if patients have significant side effects at very low doses. Recommended serum levels are 50–150 ng/ml for nortriptyline and >115 ng/ml for desipramine.

In general, TCAs are not the first antidepressant medication choice for an older patient. However, a TCA should be considered if it has worked for that individual in the past, if there are no medical contraindications, or if economic barriers to prescribing the more expensive newer medications exist. Tricyclic antidepressants may be especially helpful in patients with depression and chronic pain, such as diabetic or herpetic neuropathy.

Selective Serotonin Reuptake Inhibitors (SSRIs)

SSRIs are currently the most commonly used class of antidepressant in both younger and older adults (see Table A.2). SSRIs can usually be taken once per day, usually in the morning because they tend to be activating for most pa-

TABLE A.1 Commonly Used TCAs

Drug Name	*Unit Doses Available (in mg)*	*Therapeutic Dosage Range (mg)*	*Usual Dose (mg)*	*Usual Starting Dose (mg)*
Nortriptyline (Pamelor)	10, 25, 50, 75	25–100	25–75	10–25
Desipramine (Norpramin)	10, 25, 50, 75, 100, 150	25–200	50–100	10–25
Amitriptyline (Elavil)	10, 25, 50, 75, 100, 150	25–200	50–100	10–25
Clomipramine (Anafranil)	25, 50, 75	25–200	50–100	10–25
Imipramine (Tofranil)	10, 25, 50, 75, 100, 150	25–200	50–100	10–25
Doxepin (Adapin, Sinequan)	10, 25, 50, 75, 100, 150	25–200	50–100	10–25

tients. However, some patients can feel sedated (especially with paroxetine), and they do best taking the medication at bedtime. SSRIs have a common side effect profile, including insomnia, restlessness, agitation, fine tremor, GI distress (nausea), headache, dizziness, and sexual dysfunction. They are less likely than tricyclics to cause dry mouth, constipation, weakness, and fatigue, and are generally safe in patients with cardiac disease and in overdose. SSRIs are also indicated for patients with depression and comorbid anxiety disorders.

These medications appear to have similar efficacy, with little evidence that one is better than the others. On an individual level, however, patients may have a better response to one versus another. If a patient has a poor response to an SSRI, or is bothered by its side effects, it still makes sense to try a different SSRI.

Other Newer Antidepressants

Several other new antidepressants are available (see Table A.3). Like the SSRIs, they are relatively safe for patients with cardiac disease, are safer in overdose, and are often better tolerated than the TCAs. Bupropion (Wellbutrin) and venlafaxine (Effexor) tend to be activating and are best taken early in the day; both require multiple daily dosing. Slow-release versions of these medications

TABLE A.2 Four Commonly Used SSRIs

Drug Name	*Unit Doses Available (in mg)*	*Therapeutic Dosage Range (mg)*	*Usual Dose (mg)*	*Usual Starting Dose (mg)*
Fluoxetine (Prozac)	10, 20	10–40	10–40	10
Paroxetine (Paxil)	10, 20, 30, 40	10–40	20–40	10
Citalopram (Celexa)	20, 40, 60	10–40	20–40	10
Sertraline (Zoloft)	25, 50, 100	25-200	50-150	25

can be taken once per day (Venlafaxine XR) or twice per day (Bupropion SR). Mirtazapine (Remeron) and nefazodone (Serzone) are more sedating and best taken at bedtime. Mirtazapine is associated with increased appetite and weight gain and can be helpful for patients who have prominent loss of appetite and weight secondary to their depression. Nefazodone may require twice daily dosing.

Another antidepressant, Trazodone, is related to nefazodone but is more sedating and can cause orthostatic hypotension and priapism, a rare but serious urological emergency. Trazodone is commonly used at low doses (25–100 mg at night) to help with insomnia, either alone or in addition to other antidepressants. Its major advantage in this regard is that it does not produce dependence or impair cognitive function and coordination in the same way as benzodiazepine hypnotics. Trazodone is also an effective antidepressant, but there is a substantial risk of excessive sedation and orthostatic hypotension at the higher doses sufficient to treat major depression. For this reason, nefazodone is currently preferable to Trazodone when treating major depression.

Monoamine Oxidase Inhibitors (MAOIs)

MAOIs are an older class of antidepressant medications. They include irreversible MAOIs such as phenelzine (starting with 7.5–15 mg and increasing to 30–60 mg per day) and tranylcypromine (starting with 5–10 mg and increasing to 20–30 mg qd) and reversible MAOIs such as moclobemide (currently not available in the United States). These antidepressants are effective, in-

TABLE A.3 New Antidepressants

Drug Name	*Unit Doses Available (in mg)*	*Therapeutic Dosage Range (mg)*	*Usual Dose (mg)*	*Usual Starting Dose (mg)*	*Comments and Common Side Effects Specific to This Drug*
Bupropion[a] (Wellbutrin)	75, 100	75–150 bid–tid[b]	75–150 bid	75 qd	Twice daily dosing possible with SR preparation. Insomnia/agitation.
	SR100, SR150	100–150 bid (SR)	100–150 bid (SR)	100 qd (SR)	Avoid single doses >150 mg. Risk of seizures at high doses.
Venlafaxine (Effexor)	25, 37.5, 50, 75, 100	12.5–150 bid	25–100 bid	25 qd	Once daily dosing possible with XR preparation. Nausea, agitation, insomnia. Elevations in BP possible at higher doses.
	XR37.5 XR75 XR150	37.5–225 qd (XR)	75–225 qd (XR)	37.5 qd (XR)	
Mirtazapine (Remeron)	15, 30	7.5–45 qhs	15–30 qhs	7.5 qhs	Sedation, weight gain.
Nefazodone (Serzone)	50, 100	50–200 bid–tid	100–250 bid	50–100 bid	Sedation, GI distress. Potentially serious drug interactions with other drugs metabolized by P4503A4.

[a]Bupropion should be avoided in patients with a history of bulimia, seizures, significant head trauma, or CNS lesions that put the patient at higher risk for seizures.

[b]bid = twice daily; tid = three times daily; qhs = at bedtime; qd = per day; SR = sustained release; XR = extended release.

cluding in some patients who don't respond to other antidepressants. We will not discuss them further, however, because they are associated with significant side effects and the risk of potentially fatal hypertensive crises or serotonin syndrome. These medications also require special dietary restrictions. They are best used in consultation with a psychiatrist who is experienced in their use.

Stimulants

Stimulants such as methylphenidate (Ritalin) (starting at 5 mg in the morning and increasing to 10–20 mg twice daily) or dextroamphetamine (Dexedrine) (starting at 2.5 mg in the morning and increasing to 5–15 mg twice daily) can be helpful, both in medically ill patients who do not respond to other antidepressants and in cognitively impaired patients with pronounced apathy. At low doses, these medications cause relatively few side effects and are generally well tolerated. At higher doses, they may cause excessive activation, such as insomnia, agitation, anxiety, tremor, and anorexia, or cardiovascular side effects, such as tachycardia, arrhythmias, or hypertension. Little evidence exists for the long-term effectiveness of these medications for major depression or dysthymia. Further, a potential for addiction exists, especially in patients with prior histories of substance abuse or with long-term use.

Antidepressant Drug Interactions

All antidepressants are metabolized by the P450 isoenzyme system in the liver. Certain antidepressants inhibit specific subtypes of P450 enzymes and this may increase blood levels in patients who are taking other medications metabolized by the same isoenzyme systems. Care is advised in patients who are taking medications with a narrow therapeutic window, such as tricyclic antidepressants, digoxin, warfarin, anticonvulsants, or theophylline. They should be observed clinically for side effects and to recheck serum blood levels of such medications as the dose of the antidepressant is titrated upward. For example, patients who are taking both a tricyclic antidepressant and an SSRI should have their serum levels of the TCA checked to avoid toxicity resulting from increased TCA levels. SSRIs also are highly protein bound and may increase serum drug levels by competing for receptor sites on serum proteins.

Some of the **absolute contraindications** for combining drugs involve the combination of **nefazodone** with other drugs that are metabolized by the P450 3A4 enzyme system. For example, nefazodone should not be taken together with Seldane (terfenadine), Hismanal (astemizole), Propulsid (cisapride), Tegretol (carbamazepine), Orap (pimozide), monoamine oxidase inhibitors (MAOIs), or Halcion (triazolam). Monoamine oxidase inhibitors (MAOIs such as phenelzine or tranylcypromine) should NOT be coadministered with other antidepressants, lithium, meperidine, stimulants, pseudoephedrine, phenylephrine, reserpine, sumatriptan, l-dopa, tyramine, or morphine. Consult with a psychiatrist before using these medications as they have a narrow therapeutic window and serotonin syndrome or hypertensive crises can result if used incorrectly.

Please refer to the medication package insert, a pharmacology text, or consult with a psychiatrist or a pharmacist if you have questions about specific drug–drug interactions.

Monitoring and Managing Antidepressant Treatment

Strategies for Managing Antidepressant Side Effects

Medication side effects often lead patients to stop taking antidepressant medications. Most side effects appear early and improve over 1–2 weeks, whereas some side effects (e.g., sexual dysfunction on SSRIs) may become problematic after a few weeks of treatment. Clinicians should educate patients about side effects, ask about them during all contacts, and manage them whenever possible. The following general strategies can be helpful in addressing side effects.

- Support the patient and wait. Many side effects (e.g., GI distress with SSRIs) will subside over 1–2 weeks of treatment.
- Lower the dose of the antidepressant.
- Treat the side effects (see Table A.4).
- Change to a different antidepressant.
- Change to psychotherapy.

Switching and Discontinuing Antidepressants

Whenever possible, antidepressants should be tapered over 1–2 weeks to avoid discontinuation-related side effects. Fluoxetine is long-acting and can be discontinued abruptly, but may take 4–8 weeks to be eliminated completely.

Because all antidepressants are metabolized by the P450 cytochrome enzyme system in the liver, there is a possibility of drug interactions between two antidepressants during the period of crossover. Therefore, new antidepressants should be started at low doses during the initial 1–2 weeks to avoid unneces-

TABLE A.4 Treatment Strategies for Specific Side Effects (Other Than Changing Medications)

Side Effect	*Treatment Strategy*
Sedation	Give medication at bedtime Try stimulating coffee or tea
Orthostatic hypotension/ dizzyness	Maintain adequate hydration Get up slowly and carefully Try support hose Strongly consider changing medication
Anticholinergic (dry mouth/eyes, constipation, urinary retention, tachycardia, cognitive impairment and confusion)	Maintain adequate hydration Try sugarless gum/candy Increase dietary fiber Try artificial tears Consider bethanechol 10–20 mg bid–tid For confusion, stop medication and evaluate for delirium
GI distress/nausea	This often improves or resolves over 1-2 weeks Try to take antidepressants with meals
Activation/jitters/ tremors	Start with small doses (especially in patients with prominent anxiety symptoms or anxiety disorder) Reduce dose temporarily Consider short-term (!) trial of a benzodiazepine
Headache	Lower dose temporarily Try acetaminophen, aspirin, or NSAIDs
Insomnia	Make sure activating antidepressants are taken in A.M. Try trazodone 25–100 mg po qhs (this can cause orthostatic hypotension and priapism) Consider short-term (!) trial of a hypnotic drug
Sexual dysfunction	This may be a part of depression or an underlying medical/urological disorder Consider switch to bupropion, nefazodone, or mirtazapine, which have no known sexual side effects Decrease dose Try adding bupropion 75 mgs qhs or bid Try adding buspirone 15 mg po bid Try adding cyproheptadine 4 mg 1-2 hrs before intercourse Consider consultation with a urologist

sary side effects. Because of the slow elimination of fluoxetine (4–8 weeks), consider a longer "washout period" or very slow dose increases of new antidepressants after discontinuing fluoxetine. Wait for at least 5 weeks when starting an MAOI because of the risk of serotonin syndrome.

When the Patient Does Not Respond to a Particular Antidepressant

While the majority of patients who have a proper trial of an antidepressant improve substantially over a period of 6–12 weeks, 20–50% of patients will not respond sufficiently to the first antidepressant medication tried. Table A.5 outlines some common reasons and possible solutions for this situation.

The most important thing to remember when prescribing antidepressants is that **the medications work only if the patient takes them.** It usually takes 4–8 weeks at a therapeutic dose until patients feel some improvement in depressive symptoms. It can take as long as 12 weeks at a full therapeutic dose for depression to be substantially improved. When patients experience a remission of depressive symptoms, they need to **continue the antidepressant at full dose for at least 6–9 months** in order to prevent a relapse of depressive symptoms.

Other Medications and Special Considerations

Mood Stabilizers and Antipsychotics

Other psychotropic medications that are useful for depressed patients with bipolar disorder include antimanic agents or mood stabilizers such as lithium, valproate, or carbamazepine. In general, patients with depression due to bipolar disorder should first be treated with a mood stabilizer and only receive antidepressants if depression persists despite an adequate dose of a mood stabilizer. Some risk of inducing or worsening a manic episode exists when using antidepressant medications without the concurrent use of a mood stabilizer. It is recommended to consult a psychiatrist who is experienced in the treatment of bipolar depression when making decisions about appropriate medications for this condition.

Antipsychotic medications such as risperidone, olanazpine, quetiapine, or haloperidol can be useful for treating psychotic symptoms that may be associated with severe depressions. We recommend consultation with a psychiatrist for questions about the use of these medications.

TABLE A.5 What to Do When Patients Don't Respond to Antidepressants

Common Problem	*Possible Solution*
1. Wrong diagnosis	Reconsider diagnosis and differential diagnosis Consider anxiety, substance abuse, cognitive impairment, problems with unresolved losses or assertiveness Consider consultation with a mental health specialist
2. Insufficient dose of medication	Consider serum blood levels for TCAs Increase dose as tolerated
3. Insufficient length of treatment (Remember: it may take 6-12 weeks for patients to fully respond to antidepressants)	Support and encourage patient to stay on medication for a full trial (8-12 weeks) at a therapeutic dose—especially if there has been partial response by 4 weeks
4. Problems with adherence (Patient is not taking the medication)	Try to understand the patient's perspective, expectations, and concerns Address barriers to adherence and problem-solve together
5. Side effects (Remember: side effects may be physiological or psychological)	Wait and reassure patient. The body often gets used to the early side effects Reduce the dose (temporarily) Treat side effect(s) (see Table A.4) Change medication
6. Other complicating factors a. psychosocial stressors/ barriers b. medical problems/ medications c. psychological barriers (low self-esteem, guilt, unwillingness to let go of "sick" role) d. active alcohol or substance use e. other psychiatric problems	Address problems directly Consider consultation with a medical or mental health specialist Consider adding psychotherapy Consider additional mental health treatments as clinically indicated Consider referral to Alcoholics Anonymous or substance abuse specialty treatment if indicated
7. Treatment is not effective despite adequate trial of medication at adequate dose	Consider adding psychotherapy Consult with a geriatric psychiatrist who may recommend other treatment approaches such as augmentation of antidepressants or ECT

Antidepressant Use in Patients with Comorbid Anxiety Disorders

Many persons with depression have symptoms of anxiety, and as many as 30% may have full-blown anxiety disorders such as panic disorder or posttraumatic stress disorder. Several principles should be kept in mind when treating persons who have both depression and anxiety.

Patients with comorbid anxiety disorders can be treated with antidepressants (preferably SSRIs), which should be initiated at a low dose (e.g., 5 mg of fluoxetine or 10 mg of paroxetine) and slowly increased to full therapeutic doses as tolerated. This is because antidepressants can cause a transient worsening of anxiety symptoms before anxiety and depression respond to the treatment.

In some cases, the use of a benzodiazepine anxiolytic, such as lorazepam or clonazepam, is helpful to reduce severe anxiety during the initial weeks of treatment. However, the long-term use of such anxiolytics is strongly discouraged because they can result in sedation, worsening of depressive symptoms, cognitive and motor impairment, and psychological or physical dependence.

Antidepressant Use in Patients Who Abuse Alcohol or Other Substances

Persons with depression are at increased risk for the use of alcohol, illicit drugs, or prescription drugs. The presence of such substance use has important implications for the treatment of depression. It can reduce the person's adherence to treatments, as well as reduce the effectiveness of depression treatments. Depressed patients who misuse substances often require treatment for both problems; it is rarely sufficient to treat the depression alone. Because symptoms of depression may remit with successful treatment of the substance use problem, it is often prudent to initiate treatment for substance use before starting an antidepressant. Consult a physician who is experienced in the treatment of dually diagnosed patients if you have questions about this situation.

Herbal Remedies

Hypericum (St. John's Wort) is a plant derivative that has been shown to be well tolerated and efficacious in the treatment of mild depression but not major depression. Usual doses are 450–900 mg per day, usually in divided doses. It is not entirely clear which part of the plant contains the active ingredient responsible for its antidepressant properties. St. John's Wort is not regulated as a medication, and the content and efficacy of different commercially available preparations may vary widely. Patients who do not respond to a trial of St. John's Wort after 8–10 weeks should be strongly considered for treatment with an antidepressant medication or psychotherapy intervention. St. John's Wort has been shown to interact with a number of prescription drugs (e.g., it can decrease blood levels of antiretroviral medications used in the treatment of HIV infection). Little information exists about the safety of taking St. John's Wort in combination with other antidepressants, and we currently recommend against this practice. For these reasons, clinicians should always inquire about the use of herbal remedies during clinical interviews with depressed patients.

A number of other herbal remedies have been marketed for depression or depressive symptoms, but little scientific information about their safety or efficacy is available. Thus, we do not recommend them at this time.

Acknowledgment

Portions of this appendix have been adapted from the treatment manual for project IMPACT, a multisite treatment trial for late-life depression in primary care that is funded by the John A. Hartford Foundation and the California HealthCare Foundation (www.impact.ucla.edu). We would like to thank Wayne Katon, M.D., for his review and helpful comments on this appendix.

Appendix B: Tools for Screening and Assessment

This appendix provides a brief overview of mental health screening and assessment tools demonstrated to be reliable and valid for use with older adults. These scales are useful for screening purposes, for contributing to a comprehensive psychiatric/psychological evaluation, and for tracking progress in treatment. We review and identify sources for several clinically useful depression scales, as well as other scales that can help evaluate mental status, alcohol abuse, grief, anxiety, and dementia behavior concerns. See Appendix D for further clinical gerontology assessment resources.

Depression

Geriatric Depression Scale (GDS)

The GDS (Yesavage et al., 1983) was developed specifically for use with older adults. It excludes most somatically focused items to minimize counting symptoms that commonly overlap with medical illness (e.g., sleep disturbance, appetite changes). It also has a "yes–no" response format that is intended to minimize the cognitive demand on older adults who may have trouble considering multiple-response options on a rating scale. It may be administered as a self-report paper-and-pencil scale or through an interview format.

The GDS is a reliable and valid screening tool among community-dwelling older adults, as well as medical outpatients and inpatients, and noncognitively impaired nursing home residents (Stiles and McGarrahan, 1998). It is less useful in cases of moderate to severe dementia. As a screening tool, a score of 11 or higher is suggestive of clinically significant depression warranting further evaluation. However, to minimize identification of cases that may not really be depressed ("false positives"), a cutoff score of 14 or higher is recommended.

In addition to its use as a screening tool, the GDS is also very helpful in the context of a clinical evaluation. Administering the scale as an interview, or simply asking patients about their responses, can help to clarify what is making an individual feel helpless, worthless, bored, that life feels empty, and so forth.

Shorter versions of the GDS are commonly used. A 15-item version, developed by choosing items with the highest correlations to depression, has received the most research attention (Sheikh and Yesavage, 1986). Cutoff scores of 5, 6, or 7 are recommended in this case, depending on the study and the screening setting. Recently, a 5-item version of the scale was found to be useful in a sample of older veterans attending a geriatric outpatient medical clinic (Hoyl et al., 1999). At present, the original 30-item scale has the most research supporting its validity and is recommended when time and respondent capacity allow (Stiles and McGarrahan, 1998).

Of note, the GDS has been translated into numerous languages and its efficacy in different cultures continues to receive a fair amount of research attention. In this country, there is some concern that the GDS may not be as sensitive to depression in older African-American or Hispanic adults as compared to Caucasian elders (Baker et al., 1993; Koenig et al., 1992).

The GDS is in the public domain and appears at the end of this appendix as Table B.1. Different scale versions and translations in many languages can be accessed through the following Web site: www.stanford.edu/~yesavage/GDS.html.

Center for Epidemiological Studies Depression Scale (CES-D)

The CES-D is a self-report depression scale used extensively in community-based epidemiological research, and as a common mental health outcome measure (Radloff, 1977). The reliability and validity of the CES-D for recognizing cases of depression among older adults have received the most extensive study second to the GDS (Radloff and Teri, 1986). It is a valid screening instrument for major depression among elderly primary care patients, community-dwelling elders, and frail elders (Davidson, Feldman, and Crawford, 1994; Lyness et al., 1997; Radloff and Teri, 1986). A score of 16 or above is typically suggestive of clinical depression; for use with older adults, however, a cutoff score of 20 or above is frequently suggested to reduce false positives (Murrell, Himmelfarb, and Wright, 1983).

Although the CES-D has been found by several research groups to be valid across cultures (Gatz et al., 1993; Liang et al., 1989; McCallum et al., 1995), scale properties may differ slightly among ethnically diverse elders (Arean and Miranda, 1997) and be sensitive to language/translation issues (McCallum et al., 1995).

Shorter versions of the CES-D have also been developed and shown to be adequate depression screening tools in older adults; see, for example, Andresen et al. (1994) and Irwin, Artin, and Oxman (1999). However, different research groups report on different 10- or 11-item versions of the scale and there is not a single widely accepted shorter version of the CES-D.

The CES-D is in the public domain and appears as Table B.2.

Beck Depression Inventory (BDI)

The BDI is a commonly used self-report or interview-based depression scale, and is also used to establish baselines and outcomes in psychotherapeutic interventions for depression (Beck et al., 1979; Beck, Steer, and Garbin, 1988). The scale has 21 items, each entailing four statements about a particular symptom arranged in order of increased severity and rated from 0 to 3. Scores suggesting mild, moderate, and severe depression are 10–19, 20–30, and 31 or higher, respectively. When used as a screening tool, the BDI has been found to have adequate sensitivity and specificity for identifying depressed older adults in outpatient settings, usually using a cutoff score of 10 (see the review by Edelstein et al., 1999).

Potential problems in using the BDI with older adults are the relatively high number of somatically focused items (e.g., sleep disturbance, fatigue, loss of appetite, weight loss, somatic preoccupation, loss of libido) and the potentially challenging response style for those with mild cognitive impairment. For cognitively intact older adults, the BDI is a useful tool for tracking progress in psychotherapy.

The revised BDI-II was published in 1996, but has not yet been studied with older adults. It was developed to be consistent with DSM-IV diagnostic criteria.

The BDI and BDI-II can be obtained from the Psychological Corporation, 555 Academic Court, San Antonio, Texas, 78204, 800-872-1726, www.psychcorp.com.

Hamilton Depression Rating Scale (HDRS)

The HDRS (Hamilton, 1960) is a clinician-rated scale used in many clinical and research settings to determine the severity of depressive symptomatology. It is rated on the basis of a clinical interview. Many versions of the scale have been adapted and used in research studies (Grundy et al., 1994). A 17-item extracted

HDRS has been found to be a reliable and valid depression screening tool in elderly medical patients (Rapp, Smith, and Britt, 1990). A structured interview guide for the HDRS was published by Williams and can be adapted from this source (Williams, 1988). For use with older adults, we prefer the 24-item version, which includes cognitive symptoms of helplessness, hopelessness, and worthlessness (cited in O'Sullivan et al., 1997). Shorter versions of the HDRS are also being studied, but not specifically with older adults.

In the psychogeriatric evaluation setting, we find the HDRS to be a helpful interview guide for assessing DSM depressive symptoms. That is, the HDRS provides a structure by which to ask patients about their mood, guilt, suicidal thoughts, sleep, appetite, energy, psychomotor retardation or agitation, and interest in activity, as well as other psychiatric symptoms, including psychic and somatic anxiety, paranoid thoughts, and obsessive-compulsive symptoms. (Of note, the HDRS does not assess the individual's perceived ability to concentrate or make decisions, one of the DSM-IV symptoms for major depression.) An interview guide for the HDRS can be found in the 1988 article by J. B. W. Williams, "A Structured Interview Guide for the Hamilton Depression Rating Scale" (*Archives of General Psychiatry,* 45, 742–747).

PRIME-MD Patient Health Questionnaire (PHQ)

Though not developed or tested to date with geriatric populations specifically, this self-report version of the Primary Care Evaluation of Mental Disorders (PRIME-MD) allows for evaluation of a range of mental disorders—including depression—in the primary care setting (Spitzer et al., 1999). Further research is needed to study the PHQ's utility for diagnosing mental disorders in elderly primary care patients. The scale can be found in the 1999 article by R. L. Spitzer et al., "Validation and Utility of a Self-Report Version of the PRIME-MD: The PHQ Primary Care Study" (*Journal of the American Medical Association,* 282, 1737–1744).

Cornell Scale for Depression in Dementia

The Cornell Scale was developed as an instrument to help clinicians rate symptoms of depression in patients with dementia (Alexopoulos et al., 1988a). On the basis of information from interviews with the patient's caregiver and the patient, as well as observation of the patient, the clinician rates each of 19 items according to severity (as absent, mild or intermittent, or severe). Because individuals with dementia may have difficulty reporting on their experience of depression (due to deficits in memory, language, or insight), the other depression scales described here may not be valid for individuals with moderate to severe dementia. The Cornell Scale was not developed as a diagnostic tool, so does not have a particular cutoff score suggestive of major depression; instead, it helps to determine the severity of depressive symptoms. The Cornell scale is printed as Table B.3.

Cognitive Screening

Initial evaluation of an older adult for depression should generally include a brief cognitive screening to rule out the potential need for further cognitive evaluation (see MacNeill and Lichtenberg, 1999, for a good review of dementia screening tools). In addition to the history provided by the patient or family and behavioral observation during the interview, a brief standardized screen can give quick information about a range of cognitive domains. However, brief cognitive screening tools are NOT intended to be diagnostic for dementia or any other cognitive conditions. Further, scores on cognitive screens are strongly influenced by educational background, language, and sensory functioning, and these factors must be taken into account (Mungas et al., 1996).

The most widely used cognitive screening tool in geriatric care is the Mini-Mental State Examination (MMSE) (Folstein et al., 1975). This approximately 10-minute screen assesses orientation, immediate registration of three words, attention and calculation, short-term recall of three words, language expression, comprehension, naming, and visual construction. With a total possible score of 30 points, scores lower than 17 typically suggest severe impairment and scores from 18 to 23 suggest mild impairment (Tombaugh and McIntyre, 1992). Scores should be interpreted according to norms for age, education, and ethnicity (Crum et al., 1993).

The Modified Mini-Mental State Examination (3MS) (Teng and Chui, 1987) is an extended version of the MMSE that adds several items and allows for partial scoring of items. Added items assess verbal fluency, verbal abstraction, and delayed verbal recall. The 3MS is scored from 0 to 100, but allows for scoring the original 30-point MMSE as well. The 3MS may have improved sensitivity to Alzheimer's disease (owing to inclusion of the verbal fluency item)(Tombaugh et al., 1996) and to cognitive impairment in older stroke patients (Grace et al., 1995).

In our practice, we routinely administer the 3MS to new patients. It takes only a few minutes more than the MMSE and provides some additional clinically useful information. In particular, the use of semantic and multiple choice cues for the immediate and delayed verbal recall items provides a sense of whether memory problems appear related to deficits in encoding versus retrieval of information. The verbal fluency item is also useful, per the published report above. The 3MS is printed as Table B.4.

Alcohol Screening

A psychogeriatric evaluation should inquire about the older adult's use of alcohol and other drugs (including possible misuse of prescription medications)(Barry and Blow, 1999). The most basic part of screening for alcohol misuse, abuse, or dependence in the older adult is to ask the person if they drink alcohol and, if so, what kind, how much, how frequently, and with what consequences. Older adults who consume more than one drink daily may be at risk for negative changes in physical, cognitive, and emotional health.

The Michigan Alcoholism Screening Test–Geriatric Version (MAST-G) was developed specifically to help identify alcohol problems in older adults (Blow et al., 1992). The 24 scale items focus on the context and consequences of drinking. The scale has good sensitivity and specificity for identifying older adults with alcohol dependence (Barry and Blow, 1999). A 10-item version, the Short Michigan Alcoholism Screening Test–Geriatric Version (SMAST-G), was also developed for use in settings where time is at a premium (Barry and Blow, 1999). The MAST-G is printed as Table B.5.

Other Assessment Tools Recommended for Select Problems

Grief

The Inventory of Complicated Grief (ICG) (Prigerson et al., 1995b) is a 19-item self-report scale shown to be reliable and valid in detecting complicated grief in elderly widows and widowers. Higher scores relate to poorer functional outcomes, and the symptoms measured are distinct from the symptoms of depression. The scale is printed in:

Prigerson, H. G., Maciejewski, C. F., Reynolds, C. F., III, Bierhals, A. J., Newsom, J. T., Fasiczka, A., Frank, E., Doman, J., and Miller, M. (1995). Inventory of Complicated Grief: A scale to measure maladaptive symptoms of loss. *Psychiatry Research*, 59, 65–79.

Anxiety

The Beck Anxiety Inventory (BAI) (Beck and Steer, 1993) is a 21-item scale assessing cognitive and somatic symptoms of general anxiety; patients rate each symptom according to its distressful impact over the past week (not at all, mildly, moderately, severely). Preliminary studies have demonstrated its reliability and validity for use with older adults (Kabacoff et al., 1997; Morin et al., 1999; Wetherell and Arean, 1997), with evidence of strong internal consistency, sensible factor structures, adequate convergent and discriminant validity, and similar performance across gender and racial groups.

The BAI can be obtained from the Psychological Corporation, 555 Academic Court, San Antonio, Texas, 78204, 800-872-1726, www.psychcorp.com.

Dementia Caregiving

The Revised Memory and Behavior Problems checklist (Teri et al., 1992) is a useful scale for assessing the caregiver's perception of behavior problems in an individual with dementia, and the extent to which those problems are upsetting to the caregiver. It lists 24 potential behavioral difficulties (including memory-related problems, depression, and disruptive behaviors), each of which is rated by the caregiver in terms of its frequency of occurrence and its degree of upset to the caregiver. It is useful for planning interventions with depressed/distressed caregivers, as well as tracking the impact of interventions with the dementia patient and/or the caregiver. The scale is printed in:

Teri, L., Truax, P., Logsdon, R., Uomoto, J., Zarit, S., and Vitaliano, P. P. (1992). Assessment of behavioral problems in dementia: The revised memory and behavior problems checklist. *Psychology and Aging*, 7, 622–631.

TABLE B.1 Geriatric Depression Scale (GDS)

Choose the best answer for how you felt over the past week.

1. Are you basically satisfied with your life?	Yes	No
2. Have you dropped many of your activities and interests?	Yes	No
3. Do you feel that your life is empty?	Yes	No
4. Do you often get bored?	Yes	No
5. Are you hopeful about the future?	Yes	No
6. Are you bothered by thoughts that you can't get out of your head?	Yes	No
7. Are you in good spirits most of the time?	Yes	No
8. Are you afraid that something bad is going to happen to you?	Yes	No
9. Do you feel happy most of the time?	Yes	No
10. Do you often feel helpless?	Yes	No
11. Do you often get restless and fidgety?	Yes	No
12. Do you prefer to stay at home, rather than going out and doing new things?	Yes	No
13. Do you frequently worry about the future?	Yes	No
14. Do you feel you have more problems with memory than most?	Yes	No
15. Do you think it's wonderful to be alive now?	Yes	No
16. Do you often feel downhearted and blue?	Yes	No
17. Do you feel pretty worthless the way you are now?	Yes	No
18. Do you worry a lot about the past?	Yes	No
19. Do you find life very exciting?	Yes	No
20. Is it hard for you to get started on new projects?	Yes	No
21. Do you feel full of energy?	Yes	No
22. Do you feel that your situation is hopeless?	Yes	No
23. Do you think that most people are better off than you are?	Yes	No
24. Do you frequently get upset over little things?	Yes	No
25. Do you frequently feel like crying?	Yes	No
26. Do you have trouble concentrating?	Yes	No
27. Do you enjoy getting up in the morning?	Yes	No
28. Do you prefer to avoid social gatherings?	Yes	No
29. Is it easy for you to make decisions?	Yes	No
30. Is your mind as clear as it used to be?	Yes	No

SOURCE: Yesavage, J. A., Brink, T. L., Rose, T. L., Lum, O., Huang, V., Adey, M., and Leirer, V. O. (1983). Development and validation of a geriatric depression screening scale: A preliminary report. *Journal of Psychiatry Research*, 17, 37–49. Also: *www.stanford.edu/~yesavage/GDS.html*

TABLE B.1 (continued)

SCORING: One point for each of these answers. Cutoffs: Normal: 0–9; Mild depressives: 10–19; Severe depressives: 20–30.

1. no	6. yes	11. yes	16. yes	21. no	26. yes
2. yes	7. no	12. yes	17. yes	22. yes	27. no
3. yes	8. yes	13. yes	18. yes	23. yes	28. yes
4. yes	9. no	14. yes	19. no	24. yes	29. no
5. no	10. yes	15. no	20. yes	25. yes	30. no

NOTE: The 15-item version of the scale (Sheikh and Yesavage, 1986) includes items 1, 2, 3, 4, 7, 8, 9, 10, 12, 14, 15, 17, 21, 22, and 23.

TABLE B.2 Center for Epidemiological Studies Depression Scale (CES-D)

For each of the following statements check the box that best describes how often you have felt this way during the past week (rarely or none of the time; a little of the time; a moderate amount of the time; most or all of the time).

	Rarely or None of the Time (Less than 1 Day)	*A Little of the Time (1–2 Days)*	*A Moderate Amount of the Time (3–4 Days)*	*Most or All of the Time (5–7 Days)*
a. I was bothered by things that don't usually bother me.				
b. I did not feel like eating; my appetite was poor.				
c. I felt that I could not shake the blues, even with the help of my family or friends.				
d. I felt that I was just as good as other people.				
e. I had trouble keeping my mind on what I was doing.				
f. I felt depressed.				
g. I felt that everything I did was an effort.				
h. I felt hopeful about my future.				
i. I thought my life had been a failure.				
j. I felt fearful.				
k. My sleep was restless.				
l. I was happy.				
m. I talked less than usual.				
n. I felt lonely.				
o. People were unfriendly.				
p. I enjoyed life.				
q. I had crying spells.				
r. I felt sad.				
s. I felt that people disliked me.				
t. I could not "get going."				

SOURCE: Radloff, L. (1977). The CES-D scale: A self-report depression scale for research in the general population. *Applied Psychological Measurement*, 1, 385–401.

SCORING KEY: Rarely = 0; A little of the time = 1; A moderate amount = 2; Most of the time = 3. Reverse items d, h, l, and p, so that Rarely = 3; A little of the time = 2; A moderate amount = 1; Most of the time = 0. Sum.

TABLE B.3 Cornell Scale for Depression in Dementia

Name________________________________Age________Sex_________Date___________
Address____Telephone________________

Inpatient   Nursing Home Resident   Outpatient

Scoring System

a = unable to evaluate   1 = mild or intermittent

0 = absent   2 = severe

Ratings should be based on symptoms and signs occurring during the week prior to the interview. No score should be given if symptoms result from physical disability or illness.

A. Mood-Related Signs

1. Anxiety (anxious expression, ruminations, worrying)	a	0	1	2
2. Sadness (sad expression, sad voice, tearfulness)	a	0	1	2
3. Lack of reactivity to pleasant events	a	0	1	2
4. Irritability (easily annoyed, short tempered)	a	0	1	2

B. Behavioral Disturbance

5. Agitation (restlessness, handwringing, hairpulling)	a	0	1	2
6. Retardation (slow movements, slow speech, slow reactions)	a	0	1	2
7. Multiple physical complaints (score 0 if GI symptoms only)	a	0	1	2
8. Loss of interest (less involved in usual activities; score only if change occurred acutely; i.e., in less than 1 month)	a	0	1	2

(continues)

TABLE B.3 (continued)

C. Physical Signs				
9. Appetite loss (eating less than usual)	a	0	1	2
10. Weight loss (score 2 if greater than 5 lbs in 1 month)	a	0	1	2
11. Lack of energy (fatigues easily, unable to sustain activities; score only if changes occurred acutely, i.e. in less than one month.)	a	0	1	2
D. Cyclic Functions				
12. Diurnal variation of mood (symptoms worse in the morning)	a	0	1	2
13. Difficulty falling asleep (later than usual for this individual)	a	0	1	2
14. Multiple awakenings during sleep	a	0	1	2
15. Early morning awakening (earlier than usual for this individual)	a	0	1	2
E. Ideational Disturbance				
16. Suicide (feels life is not worth living, has suicidal wishes, or makes suicide attempt)	a	0	1	2
17. Poor self-esteem (self-blame, self-depreciation, feelings of failure)	a	0	1	2
18. Pessimism (anticipation of the worst)	a	0	1	2
19. Mood-congruent delusions (delusions of poverty, illness, or loss)	a	0	1	2

TABLE B.4 The Modified Mini-Mental State Examination (3MS)

Subject____________________ Date__________ Examiner__________

Normal or DX________________ Age______ Edu______ M F 3MS_____/100 MMS_____/30

3MS MMS

___/5 ___ DATE AND PLACE OF BIRTH

Date: year_____, month______, day______
Place: town, state____________________

___/3 ___/3 REGISTRATION
(No. of presentations:______)

SHIRT, BROWN, HONESTY
(or: SHOES, BLACK, MODESTY)
(or: SOCKS, BLUE, CHARITY)

___/7 ___/5 MENTAL REVERSAL

5 to 1
Accurate 2
1 or 2 errors/misses 0 1
DLROW
0 1 2 3 4 5

___/9 ___/3 FIRST RECALL

Spontaneous recall 3
After "Something to wear" 2
"SHIRTS, SHOES, SOCKS" 0 1

Spontaneous recall 3
After "A color" 2
"BLUE, BLACK, BROWN" 0 1

Spontaneous recall 3
After "A good personal quality" 2
"HONESTY, CHARITY, MODESTY" 0 1

___/15 ___/5 TEMPORAL ORIENTATION

Year
Accurate 8
Missed by 1 year 4
Missed by 2-5 years 0 2
Season
Accurate to within 1 month 0 1
Month
Accurate to within 5 days 2
Missed by 1 month 0 1
Day of the month
Accurate 3
Missed by 1 or 2 days 2
Missed by 3-5 days 0 1
Day of week
Accurate 0 1

___/5 ___/5 SPATIAL ORIENTATION

State 0 2
County 0 1
City (town) 0 1
Hospital/Office building/Home? 0 1

___/5 ___/2 NAMING (MMS: Pencil____, Watch____)

Forehead____, Chin____, Shoulder____
Elbow____, Knuckle____

3MS MMS

___/10 FOUR-LEGGED ANIMALS (30 seconds)
1 point each

___/6 SIMILARITIES

Arm-Leg
Body part; limb; etc. 2
Less correct answer 0 1
Laughing-Crying
Feeling; emotion 2
Other correct answer 0 1
Eating-Sleeping
Essential for life 2
Other correct answer 0 1

___/5 ___/1 REPETITION

"I WOULD LIKE TO GO HOME/OUT" 2
1 or 2 missed/wrong words 0 1
"NO IFS___ANDS___OR BUTS___"

___/3 ___/1 READ AND OBEY "CLOSE YOUR EYES"

Obeys without prompting 3
Obeys after prompting 2
Reads aloud only 0 1
(spontaneously or by request)

___/5 ___/1 WRITING (1 minute)

"(I) WOULD LIKE TO GO HOME/OUT"
(MMS: Spontaneous sentence: 0 1)

___/10 ___/1 COPYING TWO PENTAGONS (1 minute)

	Each Pentagon
5 approximately equal sides	4 4
5 unequal (>2:1) sides	3 3
Other enclosed figure	2 2
2 or more lines	0101
	Intersection
4 corners	2
Not-4-corner enclosure	0 1

___/3 ___/3 THREE STAGE COMMAND

___TAKE THIS PAPER WITH YOUR LEFT/RIGHT HAND
___FOLD IT IN HALF, AND
___HAND IT BACK TO ME

___/9 SECOND RECALL

(Something to wear) 0 1 2 3
(Color) 0 1 2 3
(Good personal quality) 0 1 2 3

SOURCE: Teng, E. L., and Chui, H. C. (1987). The Modified Mini-Mental State (3MS) Examination. *Journal of Clinical Psychiatry*, 48, 314–318.

Administration and Scoring Instructions (please see original article for further details)

Two items necessary for test administration are not printed on the form included here and can be printed on the back of the same sheet. On the reverse side, CLOSE YOUR EYES (in capital letters, approximately 1/2 inch high) can be printed on the top, and two intersecting pentagons (each side l inch long) can be drawn on the lower part, with enough space left to copy the design.

The two columns to the left of each test allow for scoring of both the 3MS and the MMSE [the original Folstein et al. (1975) Mini-Mental State Exam]. The numbers underneath each blank indicate the total number of points allowed for the 3MS and the MMSE (or MMS, as printed on the test form), respectively. (For example, the FIRST RECALL ITEM allows a total of 9 points when scored on the 3MS and 3 points when scored on the MMS.) The numbers printed to the right of the items guide partial scoring within each item.

<u>A few specific administration/scoring instructions by item:</u>

DATE AND PLACE OF BIRTH: On this item, scored only on the 3MS, assign 1 point each to the year, month, date, city or town, and state of birth.

REGISTRATION: Interviewer says, "I SHALL SAY THREE WORDS FOR YOU TO REMEMBER. REPEAT THEM AFTER I HAVE SAID ALL THREE WORDS: SHIRT . . . BROWN . . . HONESTY." The other word combinations are available to use if an individual is tested repeatedly.

MENTAL REVERSAL: In addition to asking person to spell "world" backwards (for a total of 5 points on both the 3MS and MMS), the 3MS includes a simpler, additional 2-point item (counting backward from 5); summing both items yields a total possible 7 points on the 3MS.

FIRST RECALL: Interviewer asks, "WHAT ARE THE THREE WORDS THAT I ASKED YOU TO REMEMBER?" The MMS allows only 3 points, 1 point for each word recalled (without the help of cues). The 3MS gives partial credit for correct responses with category cues (2 points per item) or multiple choice cues (1 point per item). [For example, if an individual recalled the word SHIRT with no hints (3 points), guessed the word BROWN when reminded it was a color (2 points), and could identify the word HONESTY only when given a multiple choice (1 point), the total 3MS score for this item would be 6 points.]

TEMPORAL ORIENTATION: The 3MS allows partial scoring for the year, month, and day of month items, for a total of 15 points; the MMS allows only for correct versus incorrect score (1 or 0) for all five items.

NAMING: On the 3MS, the interviewer asks the person to name each body part indicated (the interviewer points to her own forehead, chin, shoulder, elbow, knuckle) and each item is scored 1 or 0 for a total of 5 points. On the MMS, the interviewer shows a pencil and a watch and asks the person to name them, for a total of 2 points.

FOUR-LEGGED ANIMALS: The interviewer asks, "WHAT ANIMALS HAVE FOUR LEGS?" Allow 30 seconds for response, scoring for number of correct responses up to 10. This item is scored only on the 3MS, not on the MMS.

SIMILARITIES: The interviewer asks, "IN WHAT WAY ARE AN ARM AND A LEG ALIKE?" Score 0, 1, or 2 points for each of the three items, for a total of 6 possible points. Similarities is scored only on the 3MS, not on the MMS.

(continues)

Administration and Scoring Instructions (continued)

REPETITION: The interviewer says, "REPEAT WHAT I SAY, 'I WOULD LIKE TO GO HOME/OUT'." Use "home" unless the person is already at home; if so, use "out." On the 3MS only, score 0, 1, or 2 points. Then the interviewer says, "NOW REPEAT, 'NO IFS, ANDS, OR BUTS'." On the 3MS, assign 1 point each for "no ifs," "ands," "or "buts." On the MMS, score 1 or 0 for correct repetition of "no ifs, ands, or buts."

READ AND OBEY "CLOSE YOUR EYES": The interviewer holds up the paper where this command is printed and says, "PLEASE DO THIS." The 3MS allows partial scoring (0, 1, 2, or 3 points, as indicated on the form), whereas the MMS allows only for 1 or 0 points.

WRITING: For the 3MS, interviewer asks person to write the dictated sentence "I would like to go home/out." Score 1 point for each completely correct word (excluding the initial "I"). For the MMS, the person is asked to write a spontaneous sentence, scored 1 or 0.

COPYING TWO PENTAGONS: The 3MS allows for partial scoring, up to a total of 10 points, for the copy, as indicated on the form (e.g., someone who produced one 5-sided enclosed figure–4 points; and one 4-sided enclosed figure–2 points; and not intersecting–0 points, would earn a total of 6 points. The MMS allows only 1 versus 0 points, the latter if any errors in the copy.

THREE-STAGE COMMAND: The interviewer says, "TAKE THIS PAPER WITH YOUR LEFT/RIGHT (non-dominant) HAND, FOLD IT IN HALF, AND HAND IT BACK TO ME." Both 3MS and MMS assign 1 point for each step correctly done, for a total of 3 points.

SECOND RECALL: This item, scored only for the 3MS, is administered and scored as described under FIRST RECALL.

TABLE B.5 The Michigan Alcoholic Screening Test—Geriatric Version (MAST-G) © The Regents of the University of Michigan, 1991

	Yes (1)	No (0)
1. After drinking have you ever noticed an increase in your heart rate or beating in your chest?	___	___
2. When talking with others, do you ever underestimate how much you actually drink?	___	___
3. Does alcohol make you sleepy so that you often fall asleep in your chair?	___	___
4. After a few drinks, have you sometimes not eaten or been able to skip a meal because you didn't feel hungry?	___	___
5. Does having a few drinks help decease your shakiness or tremors?	___	___
6. Does alcohol sometimes make it hard for you to remember parts of the day or night?	___	___
7. Do you have rules for yourself that you won't drink before a certain time of the day?	___	___
8. Have you lost interest in hobbies or activities you used to enjoy?	___	___
9. When you wake up in the morning, do you ever have trouble remembering part of the night before?	___	___
10. Does having a drink help you sleep?	___	___
11. Do you hide your alcohol bottles from family members?	___	___
12. After a social gathering, have you ever felt embarrassed because you drank too much?	___	___
13. Have you ever been concerned that drinking might be harmful to your health?	___	___
14. Do you like to end an evening with a nightcap?	___	___
15. Did you find your drinking increased after someone close to you died?	___	___
16. In general, would you prefer to have a few drinks at home rather than go out to social events?	___	___
17. Are you drinking more now than in the past?	___	___
18. Do you usually take a drink to relax or calm your nerves?	___	___
19. Do you drink to take your mind off your problems?	___	___
20. Have you ever increased your drinking after experiencing a loss in your life?	___	___
21. Do you sometimes drive when you have had too much to drink?	___	___
22. Has a doctor or nurse ever said they were worried or concerned about your drinking?	___	___
23. Have you ever made rules about your drinking?	___	___
24. When you feel lonely, does having a drink help?	___	___

SCORING: 5 or more "yes" responses indicative of alcohol problem.

For further information, contact Frederic Blow, Ph.D., at the University of Michigan Alcohol Research Center, 400 E. Eisenhower Parkway, Suite 2A, Ann Arbor, Mich. 48108-3318, (734) 998-7952. Printed with permission from Dr. Frederic Blow.

NOTE: The Short Michigan Alcoholism Screening Test—Geriatric Version (S-MAST-G) includes items 2, 4, 5, 6, 18, 19, 20, 22, 23, and 24. A score of 2 or more suggests an alcohol problem.

Appendix C: Innovative Models of Care for Geriatric Depression

As we write this book in 2001, several exciting studies are under way to examine models of mental health care delivery to older adults. The focus of these efforts is to improve the recognition and treatment of geriatric depression in primary care settings. Although study evaluations are not yet complete, we felt it was important to alert you to these projects and encourage you to follow outcome reports in the years to come. In addition, our hope is that highlighting these models of care may help inspire program-development efforts in your own community.

Models of Mental Health/Primary Care Integration: Geriatric Focus

The Depression Clinical Specialist: Project IMPACT

Project IMPACT (Improving Mood: Promoting Access to Collaborative Treatment for Late-Life Depression) is a seven-site study in which depressed older adults will be identified in 18 primary care clinics and randomly assigned to a new disease management model for late-life depression in primary care versus care as usual. The new treatment model involves a Depression Clinical Specialist (DCS) who helps to support antidepressant treatment by the patient's primary physician, in consultation with a team psychiatrist as needed, and who can offer a 6- to 8-session course of problem-solving treatment in primary care (PST-PC)(Hegel, Barrett, and Oxman, 2000; Mynors-Wallis, 1996; Unützer et al., 2001). The DCS is usually a nurse or psychologist. Depression care is always done in cooperation with the primary care provider. The study is funded by grants from the John A. Hartford Foundation in New York, N.Y., and the California Health-Care Foundation in Oakland, Calif. See Unützer et al. (2001) or the project Web site at www.impact.ucla.edu.

Specialty Referral Versus Integrated Care: The PRISMe Study

Another study jointly funded by the Substance Abuse and Mental Health Services Administration (SAMHSA), the Veteran's Administration (VA), and the Health Resources and Services Administration (HRSA) is the Primary Care Research in Substance Abuse and Mental Health for the Elderly (PRISMe) Study. This national demonstration project is taking place in eleven sites across the country, five of which are Veterans Administration health centers. The question being studied is whether older adults with depression, anxiety, or alcohol problems are better helped if care is delivered in the primary care setting or whether it is better to refer these older adults to psychiatric specialists. The study also includes a comparison of costs between the two treatment models, as well as a calculation as to whether treating mental health and substance abuse problems leads to reduced health care costs later on. See the project Web site at www.hms.harvard.edu/aging/mhsa.

Health Specialists for Suicide Prevention: Project PROSPECT

PROSPECT (Prevention of Suicide in Primary Care Elderly Collaborative Trial) is a three-site study conducted by the National Institutes of Mental Health (NIMH) Intervention Research Centers (IRC) of Cornell University, University of Pennsylvania, and University of Pittsburgh. The intervention is offered in six primary care practices from three geographic areas (metropolitan and suburban New York, Philadelphia, and Pittsburgh) and its impact will be contrasted to that of six comparable practices offering usual care. This study is investigating the effectiveness of an intervention aimed at improving the recognition of suicidal ideation and depression by the practices and facilitating the implementation of a treatment algorithm based on the AHCPR clinical practice guidelines (Depression Guideline Panel, 1993a, 1993b). In the intervention, Health Specialists (HS) collaborate with the physicians and help them to increase recognition of depression, offer timely and appropriately targeted treatment recommendations, and encourage patients to adhere to treatment. In addition, procedures aimed at educating patients, families, and physicians on depression and suicidal ideation are implemented. The approach is expected to lead to a reduction of depressive symptomatology and suicidal ideation and behavior and to generate a practice model that has the capability to incorporate the advances of clinical science. See Bruce and Pearson (1999).

Models of Mental Health/Primary Care Integration: Adult Focus, Mixed-Age

Collaborative Management: Katon and Colleagues

Though not focusing on geriatric mental health, Katon and his colleagues (Katon et al., 1996, 1997) have published outcomes for two models of "collaborative management" designed to achieve the AHCPR guidelines for treating depression in primary care. In one model, a psychiatrist and primary care physician collaborate on prescribing antidepressants and monitoring adherence, and primary care providers receive training about the depression treatment guidelines. In another model, a psychiatrist/psychologist team collaborate in the primary care setting; a psychologist provides patient psychoeducation and brief cognitive-behavioral therapy and monitors the patient's adherence and response to medication in collaboration with a psychiatrist. The psychologist maintains close communication with the primary care physician, who makes medication adjustments based on the psychiatrist's recommendations. These collaborative interventions, studied with mostly white, middle-class adults of wide age range, showed promise for improved outcomes, cost effectiveness, and satisfaction in the treatment of major depression, with mixed results for minor depression.

Another promising approach studied by Katon's group was to target patients with poor response to antidepressant treatment initiated by the primary care physician, providing psychiatric collaboration for patients whose depressive symptoms were persisting after 6–8 weeks of treatment. The psychiatrist worked closely with the primary care physician. Patients assigned to the collaborative care model had significantly better adherence to medications, depressive outcomes, and satisfaction with care compared to those in care as usual (Katon et al., 1999).

Care Management and Feedback to Physicians: Simon and Colleagues

This study by Simon et al. (2000) examined the impact of feedback to primary care physicians about general treatment recommendations (based on a computer algorithm) for the patients they had started on antidepressant medications, alone or in combination with telephone care management with the patients. In the care management group, patients received phone calls from a care manager 8 and 16 weeks after initial prescription of the antidepressant medication. These 10- to 15-minute telephone assessments focused on current use of the medication, side effects, and severity of depressive symptoms. This information was then shared with the primary care physician along with algorithm-based treatment recommendations based on the patient's symptoms, dosage being used, and side effects reported. For example, physicians were advised to increase the dose of a medication if the patient continued to report moderate depressive symptoms and minimal side effects. The care managers also helped to schedule follow-up visits, contact patients who had discontinued treatment, and help with referrals.

The feedback and feedback plus care management conditions were compared to a usual care group. The feedback only group (without care management) showed no effect on treatment received or patient outcomes compared to usual care. The feedback plus care management intervention related to greater likelihood of receiving adequate doses of antidepressants, improvement in depression scores, lower mean depression scores on follow-up, and a lower probability of major depression at follow-up. Total health care costs did not differ significantly across the three groups.

Nurse Telehealth Care: Hunkeler and Colleagues

This study by Hunkeler et al. (2000) examined the impact of a nurse telephone intervention, alone or in combination with peer support, for primary care patients diagnosed with major depression or dysthymia who had been started on an SSRI antidepressant medication by their primary care doctor. The nurse telehealth care intervention entailed 12–14 ten-minute telephone calls during 16 weeks after enrollment. In each phone call, the nurse asked the patient about medication concerns and encouraged taking the medication regularly. In addition, the nurse provided emotional support and helped patients identify and follow up with pleasant activities. The nurse, who was part of the primary care clinic, could also address questions or concerns the patient had about their general medical health. Nurses gave regular feedback on each patient's progress to the primary care doctor.

The peer support intervention was offered in addition to the nurse telehealth intervention. Peer support was provided by health plan members who had been successfully treated for an episode of major depression or dysthymia. These volunteers were screened by a psychiatric social worker, trained, matched to patients of similar age and sex, and monitored. The peers were expected to contact patients by phone or in person for at least 6 months after the patient was enrolled in the study, with at least one contact required. It turned out that, without specific expectations for the number of contacts, most peers made only one contact and very few made face-to-face contact.

Although the nurse telehealth intervention did not appear to increase patients' adherence to their antidepressant medication (these patients had the same rates of adherence as those in the usual care group), the intervention did relate to greater reductions in depressive symptoms at 6 weeks and 6 months compared to those in usual care. The psychosocial aspect of the intervention (emotional support, monitoring behaviors) appeared to be important. The peer support did not lead to improved outcomes beyond the nurse telehealth.

Quality Improvement Programs for Depression: Wells and Colleagues

In this study by Wells et al. (2000), patients in 46 primary care clinics in six managed care organizations were screened for depressive symptoms. Clinics were randomized to usual care (practice guidelines for depression in primary care were mailed to the clinics) or to one of two Quality Improvement (QI) programs for depression (QI-medications and QI-therapy). Both QI programs entailed obtaining institutional commitment of resources to implement the program, training local experts to provide clinician education about depression care, and identifying a pool of potentially depressed patients. In the QI-medication intervention, nurse specialists provided follow-up assessment and support to encourage antidepressant medication adherence for up to 12 months. In the QI-therapy intervention, trained therapists offered cognitive-behavioral therapy for 12 to 16 sessions. Patients in both QI conditions had access to both medication and therapy. In the QI clinics, depressed patients were more likely to have had counseling or used antidepressant medication, to have seen a mental health specialist, to have had a remission of depression, and to be employed over a 12-month period.

Models of Geriatric Mental Health Care in Other Medical/Community Settings

Inpatient Medical/Surgical Screening and Care Coordination: The UPBEAT Program

This Department of Veterans Affairs clinical demonstration program (Kominski et al., 2001; Moye et al., 2001), called UPBEAT (Unified Psychogeriatric Biopsychosocial Evaluation and Treatment; P.I. Lissy Jarvik), examined the utility of conducting mental health screenings of older patients on medical and surgical units and the impact of a mental health care coordination intervention on cost, customer satisfaction, and clinical outcomes. At nine VA Medical Centers, medical/surgical inpatients over the age of 60 who were not already engaged in mental health services were approached for screening. Veterans who met screening criteria for depression, anxiety, or alcohol misuse were randomly assigned to the UPBEAT psychogeriatric care coordination program or to continued care as usual.

Veterans enrolled in the UPBEAT intervention received a comprehensive psychogeriatric assessment (usually after discharge from the hospital) that informed an individualized treatment plan addressing coordination of services (e.g., facilitating transportation to appointments, connecting elders to home care, meals, recreation, or other services in the community) and mental health concerns (e.g., psychotherapy and psychoeducation for depression, anxiety, grief, family concerns, behavioral health issues; psychopharmacology as needed). UPBEAT care coordinators were nurses, social workers, or psychologists who worked to engage sometimes reluctant patients into care, and remained available for at least the two years of the evaluation to support patients as clinical or psychosocial needs arose.

Study results show that outreach screening in medical/surgical units is a feasible way to identify older patients with previously unrecognized mental health concerns. The UPBEAT intervention led to a cost savings by reducing inpatient service utilization; thus, care coordination addressing mental health concerns may reduce inpatient bed-days of care. UPBEAT patients demonstrated high levels of satisfaction with the program.

Mobile Outreach to Seriously Mentally Ill Elderly: The PATCH Program

The PATCH (Psychogeriatric Assessment and Treatment in City Housing) study (Rabins et al., 2000) examined outreach and care provision to elderly Baltimore public housing residents with psychiatric disorders. In this model, community "gatekeepers" (building workers exposed to elders, such as janitors, groundskeepers, managers) were trained to identify elders at risk (Raschko, 1985) and refer them to a psychiatric nurse who then provided care in the residents' homes. The intervention was implemented in three buildings and compared to usual care in three other buildings. The intervention was effective in reducing psychiatric symptoms but it did not lead to a reduction in what had been called "undesirable moves" (e.g., nursing home placement, board and care placement). However, it is possible that, for some residents, such moves were clinically appropriate, whereas for other residents maintaining independent apartments was appropriate (Katz and Coyne, 2000).

Summary

The collaborative models of care being studied suggest that depression in older adults has greater hope of being recognized and treated in systems where: there is institutional commitment to integrating mental health and primary medical care services; there are structures in place not only to help screen for mental health concerns but also to support active follow-up of mental health treatments initiated; and there are mechanisms in place to address treatment nonresponse or negative side effects, and to revise treatment as needed. Several studies support the idea of a care coordinator whose job it is to follow up with and support patients' adherence to mental health interventions and to facilitate communication with primary or specialty care providers. Forthcoming study results in the next few years will clarify the models of care delivery that provide the best outcomes for older patients with depression and other mental health concerns.

Appendix D: Recommended Readings, Web Sites, and Organizational Resources

Recommended Readings

Consensus Statements and Practice Guidelines

Depression. American Psychiatric Association. (1994). Practice guideline for major depressive disorder in adults. *American Journal of Psychiatry,* 151, 625–626.

Lebowitz, B. D., Pearson, J. L., Schneider, L. S., Reynolds, C. F., III, Alexopoulos, G. S., Bruce, M. L., Conwell, Y., Katz, I. R., Meyers, B. S., Morrison, M. F., Mossey, J., Niederehe, G., and Parmalee, P. (1997). Diagnosis and treatment of depression in late life: Consensus statement update. *Journal of the American Medical Association,* 278, 1186–1190.

NIH Consensus Panel on Diagnosis and Treatment of Depression in Late Life. (1992). Diagnosis and treatment of depression in late life. *Journal of the American Medical Association,* 268, 1018–1024.

Dementia. American Psychiatric Association. (1997). Practice guideline for the treatment of patients with Alzheimer's disease and other dementias of late life. *American Journal of Psychiatry,* 154(Suppl.), 1–39.

Small, G. W., Rabins, P. V., Barry, P. P., Buckholtz, N. S., DeKosky, S. T., Ferris, S. H., Finkel, S. I., Gwyther, L. P., Khachaturian, Z. S., Lebowitz, B. D., McRae, T. D., Morris, J. C., Oakley, F., Schneider, L. S., Streim, J. E., Sunderland, T., Teri, L. A., and Tune, L. E. (1997). Diagnosis and treatment of Alzheimer disease and related disorders: Consensus statement of the American Association of Geriatric Psychiatry, the Alzheimer's Association, and the American Geriatrics Society. *Journal of the American Medical Association,* 278, 1363–1371.

Alzheimer's Association. (1998). *Guidelines for Alzheimer's disease management.* Developed by the California Workgroup on Guidelines for Alzheimer's

Disease Management in conjunction with the Los Angeles Chapter of the Alzheimer's Association. (Available at www.alzla.org)

Depression in Primary Care. Depression Guideline Panel. (1993a). *Depression in primary care: Vol. 1. Diagnosis and detection* (Clinical Practice Guideline No. 5, AHCPR Publication No. 93–0550). Rockville, Md.: Department of Health and Human Services, Public Health Service, Agency for Health Care Policy and Research. (Available at www.ahcpr.org)

Depression Guideline Panel. (1993b). *Depression in primary care: Vol. 2. Treatment of major depression* (Clinical Practice Guideline No. 5, AHCPR Publication No. 93–0551). Rockville, Md.: Department of Health and Human Services, Public Health Service, Agency for Health Care Policy and Research.

Depression Guideline Panel. (1993c). *Depression in primary care: Detection, diagnosis, and treatment: Quick reference guide for clinicians* (Clinical Practice Guideline No. 5, AHCPR Publication No. 93–0552). Rockville, Md.: Department of Health and Human Services, Public Health Service, Agency for Health Care Policy and Research.

Depression Guideline Panel. (1993d). *Depression is a treatable illness: A patient's guide* (AHCPR Publication No. 93–0553). Rockville, Md.: Department of Health and Human Services, Public Health Service, Agency for Health Care Policy and Research.

Munoz, R. F., Hollon, S. D., McGrath, E., Rehm, L. P., and VandenBos, G. R. (1994). On the AHCPR Depression in Primary Care guidelines: Further considerations for practitioners. *American Psychologist,* 49, 42–61.

Overviews on Geriatric Depression and Geriatric Mental Health

Geriatric Depression. Blazer, D. (2001). *Depression in late life,* 3rd edition. New York: Springer Publishing Company.

Schneider, L. S., Reynolds, C.F., III, Lebowitz, B. D., and Friedhoff, A. J. (Eds.). (1994). *Diagnosis and treatment of depression in late life: Results of the NIH Consensus Development Conference.* Washington, D.C.: American Psychiatric Press.

Unützer, J., Katon, W., Sullivan, M., and Miranda, J. (1999). Treating depressed older adults in primary care: Narrowing the gap between efficacy and effectiveness. *The Milbank Quarterly,* 77, 225–256.

Williamson, G. M., Shaffer, D. R., and Parmelee, P. A. (Eds.). (2000). *Physical illness and depression in older adults–A handbook of theory, research and practice* (the Plenum series in social/clinical psychology). New York: Plenum Press.

Geriatric Mental Health. U.S. Department of Health and Human Services. (1999). *Mental health: A report of the Surgeon General.* Rockville, Md.: U.S. Department of Health and Human Services, Substance Abuse and Mental Health Services Administration, Center for Mental Health Services, National Institutes of Health, National Institute of Mental Health. (See Chapter 5: Older Adults and Mental Health. Also available at www.surgeongeneral.gov/library/mentalhealth/)

American Psychological Association Working Group on the Older Adult. (1998). What practitioners should know about working with older adults. *Professional Psychology: Research and Practice,* 29, 413–427. (See on-line document at www.apa.org/pi/aging/practitioners/homepage.html)

Carstensen, L. L., Edelstein, B. A., and Dornbrand, L. (Eds.). (1996). *The practical handbook of clinical gerontology.* Thousand Oaks, Calif.: Sage Publications.

Hersen, M., and Van Hasselt, V. B. (Eds.). (1998). *Handbook of clinical geropsychology.* New York: Plenum Press.

Kennedy, G. J. (2000). *Geriatric mental health care: A treatment guide for health professionals.* New York: Guilford Publications, Inc.

Whitbourne, S. K. (Ed.). (2000). *Psychopathology in later adulthood.* New York: John Wiley & Sons.

Assessment: Clinical Gerontology

American Psychological Association. (1998). Guidelines for the evaluation of dementia and age-related cognitive decline. *American Psychologist,* 53, 1298–1303.

Baker, R., Lichtenberg, P., and Moye, J. (1998). A practice guideline for assessment of competency and capacity of the older adult. *Professional Psychology: Research and Practice,* 29, 149–154.

Green, J. (2000). *Neuropsychological evaluation of the older adult: A clinician's guidebook.* San Diego: Academic Press.

Lichtenberg, P. A. (Ed.). (1999). *Handbook of assessment in clinical gerontology.* New York: John Wiley & Sons.

U.S. Department of Veterans Affairs, National Center for Cost Containment. (1996). *Geropsychological assessment resource guide.* Milwaukee, Wisc.: Author. (Copies available from the National Technical Information Service, U.S.

Department of Commerce, 5285 Port Royal Road, Springfield, Va. 22161. Phone: 800-553-6847, Request order #PB96144365, $70.)

Psychotherapy with Older Adults

Duffy, M. (Ed.). (1999). *Handbook of counseling and psychotherapy with older adults.* New York: John Wiley & Sons.

Knight, B. G. (1996). *Psychotherapy with older adults,* 2nd edition. Thousand Oaks, Calif.: Sage Publications.

Knight, B. G. (1992). *Older adults in psychotherapy: Case histories.* Newbury Park, Calif.: Sage Publications.

Scogin, F. (2000). *The first session with seniors: A step-by-step guide.* San Francisco: Jossey-Bass Publishers.

Zarit, S. H., and Knight, B. G. (Eds.). (1996). *A guide to psychotherapy and aging: Effective clinical interventions in a life-stage context.* Washington, D.C.: American Psychological Association.

Treatment Manuals/Guides

Cognitive-Behavioral Psychotherapy. Thompson, L. W., Gallagher-Thompson, D., and Dick, L. P. (1995). *Cognitive-behavioral therapy for late life depression: A therapist manual.* Palo Alto, Calif.: Older Adult and Family Center, Veterans Affairs Palo Alto Health Care System.

Dick, L. P., Gallagher-Thompson, D., Coon, D. W., Powers, D. V., and Thompson, L. W. (1995). *Cognitive-behavioral therapy for late life depression: A client manual.* Palo Alto, Calif.: Older Adult and Family Center, Veterans Affairs Palo Alto Health Care System.

CBT Self-Help Guides. Burns, D. (1980). *Feeling good.* New York: Guilford Press.

Lewinsohn, P. M., Munoz, R., Youngren, M., and Zeiss, A. (1986). *Control your depression.* Englewood Cliffs, N.J.: Prentice Hall.

Interpersonal Psychotherapy. Weissman, M. M., Markowitz, J. C., and Klerman, G. L. (2000). *Comprehensive guide to interpersonal psychotherapy.* New York: Basic Books.

Problem-Solving Therapy. Nezu, A. M., Nezu, C. M., and Perri, M. G. (1989). *Problem-solving therapy for depression: Theory, research, and clinical guidelines.* New York: John Wiley & Sons.

Psychopharmacology

Arana, G. W., and Rosenbaum, J. F. (2000). *Handbook of psychiatric drug therapy.* Philadelphia: Lippincott Williams & Wilkins.

Salzman, C. (1997). *Clinical geriatric psychopharmacology.* 3rd edition. Baltimore: Williams & Wilkins.

Comorbid Psychogeriatric Issues

Suicide in Late Life. Kennedy, G. J. (Ed.). (1996). *Suicide and depression in late life: Critical issues in treatment, research, and public policy.* New York: John Wiley & Sons.

McIntosh, J. L., Santos, J. F., Hubbard, R. W., and Overholser, J. C. (1994). *Elder suicide: Research, theory, and treatment.* Washington, D.C.: American Psychological Association.

Pearson, J. L., and Brown, G. K. (2000). Suicide prevention in late life: Direction for science and practice. *Clinical Psychology Review,* 20, 685–705.

Richman, J. (1993). *Preventing elderly suicide: Overcoming personal despair, professional neglect, and social bias.* New York: Springer Publishing Company.

Steffens, D. C., and Blazer, D. G. (1999). Suicide in the elderly. In D. G. Jacobs (Ed.), *The Harvard Medical School guide to suicide assessment and intervention* (pp. 443–462). San Francisco: Jossey-Bass Publishers.

Dementia and Depression. Katz, I. R. (1998). Diagnosis and treatment of depression in patients with Alzheimer's disease and other dementias. *Journal of Clinical Psychiatry,* 59(Suppl. 9), 38–44.

Rosenstein, L. D. (1998). Differential diagnosis of the major progressive dementias and depression in middle and late adulthood: A summary of the literature of the early 1990s. *Neuropsychology Review,* 8, 109–167.

Storandt, M., and VandenBos, G. R. (Eds.). (1995). *Neuropsychological assessment of dementia and depression in older adults: A clinician's guide.* Washington, D.C.: American Psychological Association.

Help for Dementia Caregivers. Gallagher-Thompson, D., Rose, J., Florsheim, M., Gantz, F., Jacome, P., Dalmaestro, S., Peters, L., Arguello, D., Johnson, C., Moorehead, R. S., Polich, T. M., Chesney, M., and Thompson, L. W. (1992). *Controlling your frustration: A class for caregivers.* Palo Alto, Calif.: Department of Veterans

Affairs Medical Center. (To order, call 650-723-7063; Stanford Geriatric Education Center, 703 Welch Road, Suite H1, Stanford, Calif. 94305. Or see the Web site www.stanford.edu/dept/medfm/gec/page1.html)

Mace, N. L., Rabins, P. V., and McHugh, P. R. (1999). *The 36-hour day: A family guide to caring for persons with Alzheimer disease, related dementing illnesses, and memory loss in later life,* 3rd edition. Baltimore: Johns Hopkins University Press.

Rabins, P. V., Lyketsos, C. G., and Steele, C. (1999). *Practical dementia care.* Oxford: Oxford University Press.

Anxiety Disorders. Beck, J. G., and Stanley, M. A. (1997). Anxiety disorders in the elderly: The emerging role of behavior therapy. *Behavior Therapy,* 28, 83–100.

Ruskin, P. E., and Talbott, J. A. (Eds.). (1996). *Aging and posttraumatic stress disorder.* Washington, D.C.: American Psychiatric Press.

Stanley, M. A., and Beck, J. G. (2000). Anxiety disorders. *Clinical Psychology Review,* 20, 731–754.

Wetherell, J. L. (1998). Treatment of anxiety in older adults. *Psychotherapy,* 35, 444–458.

Bereavement. Rosenzweig, A., Prigerson, H., Miller, M. D., and Reynolds, C. F., III. (1997). Bereavement and late-life depression: Grief and its complications in the elderly. *Annual Review of Medicine,* 48, 421–428.

Zisook, S., and Schuchter, S. R. (1996). Grief and bereavement. In J. Sadavoy, L. W. Lazarus, L. F. Jarvik, and G. T. Grossberg (Eds.), *Comprehensive review of geriatric psychiatry,* 2nd edition. Washington, D.C.: American Psychiatric Press.

Alcohol Problems. Barry, K. L., Oslin, D. W., and Blow, F. C. (2001). *Alcohol problems in older adults: Prevention and management.* New York: Springer Publishing Company.

Center for Substance Abuse Treatment. (1998). *Treatment improvement protocol #26: Substance abuse among older adults* (DHHS Publication No. (SMA) 98-3179). Rockville, Md.: Department of Health and Human Services.

Personality Disorders. Rosowsky, E., Abrams, R. C., and Zweig, R. A. (Eds.). (1999). *Personality disorders in older adults: Emerging issues in diagnosis and treatment.* Mahwah, N.J.: Lawrence Erlbaum Associates.

Ethnic Diversity

Haley, W. E., Han, B., and Henderson, J. N. (1998). Aging and ethnicity: Issues for clinical practice. *Journal of Clinical Psychology in Medical Settings*, 5, 393–409.

Padgett, D. K. (Ed). (1995). *Handbook on ethnicity, aging, and mental health.* Westport, Conn.: Greenwood Press.

Tsai, J. L., and Carstensen, L. L. (1996). Clinical intervention with ethnic minority elders. In L. L. Carstensen, B. A. Edelstein, and L. Dornbrand (Eds.), *The practical handbook of clinical gerontology* (pp. 76–106). Thousand Oaks, Calif.: Sage Publications.

The Standford Geriatric Education Center (SGEC): See Web site at www.stanford.edu/dept/medfm/gec/page1.html

From the Web site's homepage: "The Stanford Geriatric Education Center provides a variety of ethnogeriatric programs and curriculum resource materials to educate health care professionals on the cultural issues associated with aging and health. The SGEC promotes cultural sensitivity and cultural competence to improve the quality of health care delivered to the rapidly growing population of ethnic minority elders in the United States."

Medical Issues

Beers, M. H., and Berkow, R. (2000). *The Merck manual of geriatrics,* 3rd edition. Whitehouse Station, N.J.: Merck & Co, Inc. Available at www.merck.com/pubs/mm_geriatrics/

Miller, K. E., Zylstra, R. G., and Standridge, J. B. (2000). The geriatric patient: A systematic approach to maintaining health. *American Family Physician,* 61, 1089–1104.

Williams, M. E. (1995). *The American Geriatrics Society's complete guide to aging and health.* New York: Harmony Books.

Long-Term Care

Conn, D., Hermann, N., Kaye, A., Rewilak, D., and Schogt, B. (Eds). *Practical psychiatry in the long-term care facility: A handbook for staff,* 2nd edition. Seattle: Hogrefe & Huber Publishers.

Lichtenberg, P. A., Smith, M., Frazer, D., et al. (1998). Standards for psychological services in long-term care facilities. *The Gerontologist,* 38, 122–127.

Molinari, V. (Ed.). (2000). *Professional psychology in long term care: A comprehensive guide.* New York: Hatherleigh Press.

Rubinstein, R. L., and Lawton, M. P. (Eds.). (1997). *Depression in long term and residential care: Advances in research and treatment.* New York: Springer Publishing Company.

Teams

Clark, P. G. (1997). Values in health care professional socialization: Implications for geriatric education in interdisciplinary teamwork. *The Gerontologist,* 37, 441–451.

Counsell, S. R., Kennedy, R. D., Szwabo, P., Wadsworth, N. S., and Wohlgemuth, C. (1999). Curriculum recommendations for resident training in geriatrics interdisciplinary team care. *Journal of the American Geriatrics Society,* 47, 1145–1148.

Qualls, S. H., and Czirr, R. (1988). Geriatric health teams: Classifying models of professional and team functioning. *The Gerontologist,* 28, 372–376.

Zeiss, A. M., and Steffen, A. M. (1996). Interdisciplinary health care teams: The basic unit of care. In L. L. Carstensen, B. A. Edelstein, and L. Dornbrand (Eds.), *The practical handbook of clinical gerontology.* Thousand Oaks, Calif.: Sage Publications.

Training in the Field

American Psychological Association. (2000). *Training guidelines for practice in clinical geropsychology: Report of the APA Interdivisional Task Force on Qualifications for Practice in Clinical and Applied Geropsychology, Draft #8.* Washington, D.C.: APA. Available at aging.ufl.edu/apadiv20/qualtf8b.htm

Gatz, M., and Finkel, S. I. (1995). Education and training of mental health service providers. In M. Gatz (Ed.), *Emerging issues in mental health and aging* (pp. 282–302). Washington, D.C.: American Psychological Association.

Jeste, D. V., Alexopoulos, G. S., Bartels, S. J., Cummings, J. L., Gallo, J. J., Gottlieb, G. L., Halpain, M. C., Palmer, B. W., Patterson, T. L., Reynolds, C. F., III, and Lebowitz, B. D. (1999). Consensus statement on the upcoming crisis in geriatric mental health care: Research agenda for the next 2 decades. *Archives of General Psychiatry,* 56, 848–852.

Knight, B., Teri, L., Wohlford, P., and Santos, J. (Eds) (1995). *Mental health services for older adults.* Washington, D.C.: American Psychological Association.

Also, see listing for Council on Social Work Education (CSWE) below regarding an initiative for gerontology education for social workers.

Geriatric Mental Health Service Delivery

Gatz, M. (Ed.). (1995). *Emerging issues in mental health and aging.* Washington, D.C.: American Psychological Association.

Gatz, M., and Smyer, M. (1992). The mental health system and older adults in the 1990s. *American Psychologist,* 47, 741–751.

Gatz, M., and Smyer, M. A. (2001). Mental health and aging at the outset of the twenty-first century. In J. E. Birren and K. W. Schaie. *Handbook of the psychology of aging,* 5th edition (pp. 523–544). San Diego: Academic Press.

Hartman-Stein, P. E. (Ed.). (1998). *Innovative behavioral healthcare for older adults: A guidebook for changing times.* San Francisco: Jossey-Bass Publishers.

Norris, M. P., Molinari, V., and Rosowsky, E. (1998). Providing mental health care to older adults: Unraveling the maze of Medicare and managed care. *Psychotherapy,* 35, 490–497.

Useful Web Sites

Administration on Aging (AOA): www.aoa.dhhs.gov

Rich source of information for providers and consumers about policy updates, aging services, connections to local Area Agencies on Aging. Also, "Eldercare Locator" number 800-677-1116, a general information and referral service that connects consumers to local agencies. Fact sheets on many health- and policy-related issues.

National Institute of Aging (NIA), Health Information: www.nih.gov/nia/health/

Section of the NIA Web site devoted to health information and resources for consumers and professionals. "Age-pages" can be printed with information on a wide range of geriatric health, mental health, and social concerns (e.g., crime, driving, long-term care planning) for patient/family education. Access to Alzheimer's Disease Education and Referral (ADEAR) services.

National Institutes of Mental Health (NIMH): www.nimh.nih.gov

Information for researchers, professionals, and consumers regarding latest research. Can order "fact sheets" on a range of mental health issues for patient education purposes.

Agency for Healthcare Research and Quality (AHRQ): www.ahcpr.gov/

AHRQ supports research that provides evidence-based information on health care outcomes, quality, cost, use, and access. Information is available to help patients and clinicians, as well as health system leaders, make informed decisions about health care services. The Web site provides access to research outcome data and previously published clinical practice guidelines (including guidelines for assessing and treating depression in primary care) and consumer versions of these.

Medicare: www.medicare/gov

Information about Medicare coverage, policy managed care plans, Medigap supplemental insurance policies, contact numbers relevant for both consumers and providers, and information about choosing nursing homes.

Social Security Administration: www.ssa.gov

Information on benefits, frequently asked questions, and local contact phone numbers.

Department of Veterans Affairs (DVA): www.va.gov

Information on veterans' benefits and services. Many older adults served in the military and may not be aware of health care and other services available through the DVA.

National Center on Elder Abuse (NCEA): www.elderabusecenter.org/

Information for providers, consumers, and researchers on elder abuse statistics, research, laws, reporting guidelines and contacts.

Firstgov for seniors: www.seniors.gov

This Web site, created and maintained by the Social Security Administration, helps users to access all government sites that provide services for senior citizens, such as the SSA, Health Care Financing Administration, Administration on Aging, and Department of Veterans Affairs. The site provides links to all federal agencies and 50 states.

Sensitizing People to the Process of Aging: A simulation: fcs.tamu.edu/aging/SENSORY.HTM

This Web site provides easy-to-use exercises to increase sensitivity to the aging process (e.g., changes in sight, hearing, taste, dexterity, touch, taste, smell, mobility, and balance).

McArthur Foundation Toolkit for the Management of Depression in Primary Care: www.depression-primarycare.org/

This Web site was developed to provide primary care providers with informational and educational resources to improve care of depression in primary care.

Quality Improvement Materials from Partners in Care: www.rand.org/publications/MR/MR1198/

This Web site provides many resources for implementing the Partners in Care approach to treating depression in primary care, with training, informational, and patient education materials regarding medication and psychotherapy, developed for socioeconomically and ethnically diverse populations.

Canadian Internet Mental Health Information: www.mentalhealth.com/fr20.html

This Web site compiles information about diagnosis, treatment, and research regarding a wide range of mental disorders.

Organizational Resources

Professional Organizations

American Society on Aging (ASA)–a multidisciplinary organization focused on practice, with an emphasis on education and training

833 Market Street, Suite 511
San Francisco, Calif. 94103–1824
(415) 974–9600
www.asaging.org

The Gerontological Society of America (GSA)–a multidisciplinary organization focused on promotion and dissemination of research on aging

1030 15th Street, NW, Suite 250
Washington, D.C. 20005
(202) 842–1275
www.geron.org

American Geriatrics Society (AGS)–initially for geriatric physicians, now a multidisciplinary organization promoting research, education, practice, and policy in geriatric care

The Empire State Building
250 Fifth Avenue, Suite 801
New York, N.Y. 10118
(212) 308–1414
www.americangeriatrics.org/

American Association for Geriatric Psychiatry (AAGP)

7910 Woodmont Avenue, Suite 1050
Bethesda, Md. 20814
(301) 654–7850
www.aagpgpa.org

American Psychological Association (APA)–division on Adult Development and Aging, and a Clinical Geropsychology section within Clinical Psychology division (see the Web site)

750 First Street, NE
Washington, D.C. 20002–4242
(800) 374–2721, (202) 336–5500
www.apa.org/

For Clinical Geropsychology: bama.ua.edu/~appgero/apa12_2/
For Adult Development and Aging: aging.ufl.edu/apadiv20/apadiv20.htm

National Association of Social Workers (NASW)–Section on Aging (see the Web site)
750 First Street, NE, Suite 700
Washington, D.C. 20002–4241
(800) 638–8799, (202) 408–8600
www.naswdc.org/

Council on Social Work Education (CSWE)–Strengthening Aging and Gerontology Education for Social Work (SAGE-SW) program to develop curriculum and training materials for social work education in gerontology
1725 Duke Street, Suite 500
Alexandria, Va. 22314–3457
(703) 683–8080
www.cswe.org/

National Gerontological Nursing Association (NGNA)
7794 Grow Drive
Pensacola, Fla. 32514
(850) 473–1174
www.ngna.org/

National Association of Professional Geriatric Care Managers (GCM)
1604 N. Country Club Road
Tucson, Ariz. 85716–3102
(520) 881–8008
www.caremanager.org

Advocacy/Consumer Organizations

Alzheimer's Association
919 North Michigan Avenue
Suite 1100
Chicago, Ill. 60611–1676
(800) 272–3900
www.alz.org/

This Web site has information for patients, family caregivers, professionals, and researchers regarding Alzheimer's disease and services.

American Association of Retired Persons (AARP)
601 E St., NW
Washington, D.C. 20049
(800) 424–3410
www.aarp.org

AARP serves the needs and interests of people age 50 and older through information and education, advocacy, and community services. The Web site is a rich resource for a wide range of health, financial, political, and other information of interest to older adults.

National Alliance for the Mentally Ill (NAMI)
Colonial Place Three
2107 Wilson Blvd., Suite 300
Arlington, Va. 22201–3042
(800) 950-NAMI, (703) 524–7600
www.nami.org

National Depressive and Manic Depressive Association (NDMDA)
730 N. Franklin, Suite 501
Chicago, Ill. 60601
(800) 826–3632, (312) 642–0049
www.ndmda.org

National Foundation for Depressive Illness, Inc.
P.O. Box 2257
New York, N.Y. 10116
(800) 239–1265, (202) 268–4260
www.depression.org

National Mental Health Association (NMHA)
1021 Prince Street
Alexandria, Va. 22314–2971
(800) 969–6642, (703) 684–7722
www.nmha.org

References

Adams, W., Barry, K. L., and Fleming, M. F. (1996). Screening for alcohol use in older primary care patients. *Journal of the American Medical Association, 279*, 1964–1967.

Alexopoulos, G. S., Abrams, R. C., Young, R. C., and Shamoian, C. A. (1988a). Cornell Scale for Depression in Dementia. *Biological Psychiatry,* 23, 271–284.

Alexopoulos, G. S., Young, R. C., Meyers, B. S., Abrams, R. C., and Shamoian, C. A. (1988b). Late-onset depression. *Psychiatric Clinics of North America,* 11, 101–115.

Alexopoulos, G. S., Meyers, B. S., Young, R. C., Campbell, S., Silbersweig, D., and Charlson, M. (1997). "Vascular depression" hypothesis. *Archives of General Psychiatry,* 54, 915–922.

Alexopoulos, G. S., Meyers, B. S., Young, R. C., Kalayam, B., Kakuma, T., Gabrielle, M., Sirey, J. A., and Hull, J. (2000). Executive dysfunction and long-term outcomes of geriatric depression. *Archives of General Psychiatry,* 57, 285–290.

American Psychiatric Association. (1994). *Diagnostic and statistical manual of mental disorders,* 4th edition. Washington, D.C.: American Psychiatric Association.

Andresen, E. M., Malmgren, J. A., Carter, W. B., and Patrick, D. L. (1994). Screening for depression in well older adults: Evaluation of a short from of the CES-D. *American Journal of Preventive Medicine,* 10, 77–84.

Archbold, P. G., Steward, B. J., Greenlick, M. R., and Harvath, T. A. (1992). The clinical assessment of mutuality and preparedness in family caregivers to frail older people. In S. G. Funk, E. M. Tornquist, M. T. Champagne, and R. A. Weise (Eds.), *Key aspects of elder care: Managing falls, incontinence, and cognitive impairment.* New York: Springer Publishing Co.

Arean, P. A., and Miranda, J. (1997). The utility of the Center for Epidemiological Studies-Depression Scale in older primary care patients. *Aging and Mental Health,* 1, 47–56.

Ariyo, A. A., Haan, M., Tangen, C. M., Rutledge, J. C., Cushman, M., Dobs, A., and Furberg, C. D., for the Cardiovascular Health Study Collaborative Research Group. (2000). Depressive symptoms and risks of coronary heart disease and mortality in elderly Americans. *Circulation,* 102, 1773–1779.

Baker, F. M., Espino, D. V., Robinson, B. H., and Stewart, B. (1993). Depression among elderly African Americans and Mexican Americans. *American Journal of Psychiatry,* 150, 987–988.

Ballenger, J. C., Davidson, J. R. T., Lecrubier, Y., Nutt, D. J., Foa, E. B., Kessler, R. C., and McFarlane, A. C. (2000). Consensus statement on posttraumatic stress disorder from the international consensus group on depression and anxiety. *Journal of Clinical Psychiatry,* 61, 60–66.

Barry, K. L., and Blow, F. (1999). Screening and assessment of alcohol problems in older adults. In P. A. Lichtenberg (Ed.), *Handbook of assessment in clinical gerontology* (pp. 243–269). New York: John Wiley & Sons.

Bartels, S. J., Horn, S., Sharkey, P., and Levine, K. (1997). Treatment of depression in older primary care patients in health maintenance organizations. *International Journal of Psychiatry in Medicine,* 27, 215–231.

Beck, A. T., and Steer, R. A. (1993). *Beck Anxiety Inventory manual,* 2nd edition. San Antonio, Texas: Psychological Corporation.

Beck, A. T., Rush, A. J., Shaw, B. F., and Emery, G. (1979). *Cognitive therapy of depression.* New York: Guilford Press.

Beck, A. T., Steer, R. A., and Garbin, M. G. (1988). Psychometric properties of the Beck Depression Inventory: Twenty-five years of evaluation. *Clinical Psychology Review,* 8, 77–100.

Beck, J. G., and Stanley, M. A. (1997). Anxiety disorders in the elderly: The emerging role of behavior therapy. *Behavior Therapy,* 28, 83–100.

Beekman, A. T. F., Deeg, D. J. H., van Tilburg, T., Smit, J. H., Hooijer, C., and van Tilburg, W. (1995). Major and minor depression in later life: A study of prevalence and risk factors. *Journal of Affective Disorders,* 36, 65–75.

Blake, D., Weathers, F., Nagy, L., Kaloupek, D., Klauminzer, G., Charney, D., and Keane, T. (1995). The development of a Clinician-Administered PTSD Scale. *Journal of Traumatic Stress,* 8, 75–90.

Blazer, D., Hughes, D. C., and Fowler, N. (1989). Anxiety as an outcome symptom of depression in elderly and middle-aged adults. *International Journal of Geriatric Psychiatry,* 4, 273–278.

Blazer, D. G. (1994). Epidemiology of late-life depression. In L. S. Schneider, C. F. Reynolds III, B. D. Lebowitz, and A. J. Friedhoff (Eds.), *Diagnosis and treatment of depression in late life: Results of the NIH Consensus Development Conference* (pp. 9–19). Washington, D.C.: American Psychiatric Press.

Blazer, D. G., and Koenig, H. G. (1996). Mood disorders. In E. W. Busse and D. G. Blazer (Eds.), *The American Psychiatric Press Textbook of Geriatric Psychiatry,* 2nd edition (pp. 235–263). Washington, D.C.: American Psychiatric Press.

Block, S. D., and Billings, J. A. (1995). Patient requests for euthanasia and assisted suicide in terminal illness: The role of the psychiatrist. *Psychosomatics,* 36, 445–457.

Blow, F. C., Brower, K. J., Schulenberg, J. E., Demo-Dananberg, L. M., Young, J. P., and Beresford, T. P. (1992). The Michigan Alcoholism Screening Test-Geriatric Version (MAST-G): A new elderly-specific screening instrument. *Alcoholism: Clinical and Experimental Research,* 16, 372.

Breitbart, W., Rosenfeld, B., Pessin, H., Kaim, M., Funesti-Esch, J., Galietta, M., Nelson, C. J., and Brescia, R. (2000). Depression, hopelessness, and desire for hastened death in terminally ill patients with cancer. *Journal of the American Medical Association,* 284, 2907–2911.

Brennan, P. L., and Moos, R. H. (1996). Late-life problem drinking: Personal and environmental risk factors for 4-year functioning outcomes and treatment seeking. *Journal of Substance Abuse,* 8, 167–180.

Brody, C. M. (1999). Existential issues of hope and meaning in late life therapy. In M. Duffy (Ed.), *Handbook of counseling and psychotherapy with older adults* (pp. 91–106). New York: John Wiley & Sons.

Bruce, M. L., and Pearson, J. L. (1999). Designing an intervention to prevent suicide: Prevention of suicide in primary care elderly collaborative trial (PROSPECT). *Dialogues in Clinical Neuroscience,* 1, 100–112.

Bruce, M. L., Seeman, T. E., Merrill, S. S., and Blazer, D. G. (1994). The impact of depressive symptomatology on physical disability: MacArthur Studies of Successful Aging. *American Journal of Public Health,* 84, 1796–1799.

Callahan, C. M., Hui, S. L., Nienaber, N. A., Musick, B. S., and Tierney, W. M. (1994). Longitudinal study of depression and health services use among elderly primary care patients. *Journal of the American Geriatrics Society,* 42, 833–838.

Callahan, C. M., Hendrie, H. C., Nienaber, N. A., and Tierney, W. M. (1996). Suicidal ideation among older primary care patients. *Journal of the American Geriatrics Society,* 44, 1205–1209.

Callahan, E. J., Bertakis, K. D., Azari, R., Robbins, J. A., Helms, L. J., and Chang, D. W. (2000). The influence of patient age on primary care resident physician–patient interaction. *Journal of the American Geriatrics Society,* 48, 30–35.

Center for Substance Abuse Treatment. (1998). *Treatment improvement protocol #26: Substance abuse among older adults* (DHHS Publication No. (SMA) 98-3179). Rockville, Md.: Department of Health and Human Services.

Chambliss, D. L., Sanderson, W. C., Shoham, V., Johnson, S. B., Pope, K. S., Crits-Christoph, P., Baker, M., Johnson, B., Woody, S. R., Sue, S., Beutler, L., Williams, D. A., and McCurry, S. (1996). An update on empirically validated therapies. *The Clinical Psychologist,* 49, 5–18.

Clipp, E. C., and Elder, J., G.H. (1996). The aging veteran of World War II. In P. E. Ruskin and J. A. Talbott (Eds.), *Aging and posttraumatic stress disorder* (pp. 19–51). Washington, D.C.: American Psychiatric Press.

Conwell, Y. (1994). Suicide in elderly patients. In L. S. Schneider, C. F. Reynolds III, B. D. Lebowitz, and A. J. Friedhoff (Eds.), *Diagnosis and treatment of depression in late life* (pp. 397–418). Washington, D.C.: American Psychiatric Press.

Conwell, Y., Duberstein, P. R., Cox, C., Hermann, J. H., Forbes, N. T., and Caine, E. D. (1996). Relationships of age and axis I diagnoses in victims of completed suicide: A psychological autopsy study. *American Journal of Psychiatry,* 153, 1001–1008.

Conwell, Y., Lyness, J. M., Duberstein, P., Cox, C., Seidlitz, L., DiGiorgio, A., and Caine, E. D. (2000). Completed suicide among older patients in primary care practices: A controlled study. *Journal of the American Geriatrics Society,* 48, 23–29.

Coon, D. W., Rider, K., Gallagher-Thompson, D., and Thompson, L. (1999). Cognitive-behavioral therapy for the treatment of late-life distress. In M. Duffy (Ed.), *Handbook of counseling and psychotherapy with older adults* (pp. 487–510). New York: John Wiley & Sons.

Crum, R. M., Anthony, J. C., Bassett, S. S., and Folstein, M. F. (1993). Population-based norms for the Mini-Mental State Examination by age and education level. *Journal of the American Medical Association, 269*, 2386–2391.

Cummings, N. A. (1998). Approaches to preventive care. In P. E. Hartman-Stein (Ed.), *Innovative behavioral healthcare for older adults: A guidebook for changing times* (pp. 1–17). San Francisco: Jossey-Bass Publishers.

Davidson, H., Feldman, P. H., and Crawford, S. (1994). Measuring depressive symptoms in the frail elderly. *Journal of Gerontology, 49*, P159-P164.

Devanand, D. P., Nobler, M. S., Singer, T., Kiersky, J. E., Turret, N., Roose, S. P., and Sackeim, H. A. (1994). Is dysthymia a different disorder in the elderly? *American Journal of Psychiatry,* 151, 1592–1599.

Dupree, L. W., and Schonfeld, L. (1999). Management of alcohol abuse in older adults. In M. Duffy (Ed.), *Handbook of counseling and psychotherapy with older adults* (pp. 632–649). New York: John Wiley & Sons.

Edelstein, B., Kalish, K. D., Drozdick, L. W., and McKee, D. R. (1999). Assessment of depression and bereavement in older adults. In P. A. Lichtenberg (Ed.), *Handbook of assessment in clinical gerontology.* New York: John Wiley & Sons.

Ferrell, B. R., and Ferrell, B. A. (Eds.). (1996). *Pain in the elderly.* Seattle: IASP Press.

Finkel, S. I. (1991). Group psychotherapy in later life. In W. A. Myers (Ed.), *New techniques in the psychotherapy of older patients* (pp. 223–244). Washington, D.C.: American Psychiatric Press.

Fiske, A., Kasl-Godley, J. E., and Gatz, M. (1998). Mood disorders in late life. In B. Edelstein (Ed.), *Clinical geropsychology* (Vol. 7, pp. 193–229). New York: Elsevier.

Fleming, M. F., Manwell, L. B., Barry, L., Adams, W., and Stauffacher, E. A. (1999). Brief physician advice for alcohol problems in older adults: A randomized community-based trial. *Journal of Family Practice,* 48, 378–384.

Flint, A. J. (1994). Epidemiology and comorbidity of anxiety disorders in the elderly. *American Journal of Psychiatry,* 151, 640–649.

Flint, A. J., and Rifat, S. L. (1998a). The treatment of psychotic depression in later life: A comparison of pharmacotherapy and ECT. *International Journal of Geriatric Psychiatry,* 13, 23–28.

Flint, A. J., and Rifat, S. L. (1998b). Two-year outcome of psychotic depression in late life. *American Journal of Psychiatry,* 155, 178–183.

Folstein, M. F., Folstein, S. E., and McHugh, P. R. (1975). "Mini-Mental State." A practical method for grading the cognitive state of patients for the clinician. *Journal of Psychiatric Research,* 12, 189–198.

Forsell, Y., Jorm, A. F., and Winblad, B. (1994). Association of age, sex, cognitive dysfunction, and disability with major depressive symptoms in an elderly sample. *American Journal of Psychiatry,* 151, 1600–1604.

Frasure-Smith, N., Lesperance, F., and Talajic, M. (1993). Depression following myocardial infarction: Impact on 6-month survival. *Journal of the American Medical Association,* 270, 1819–1825.

Gallagher-Thompson, D., and DeVries, H. M. (1994). "Coping with frustration" classes: Development and preliminary outcomes with women who care for relatives with dementia. *The Gerontologist,* 34, 548–552.

Gallagher-Thompson, D., and Thompson, L. W. (1996). Applying cognitive-behavioral therapy to the psychological problems of later life. In S. H. Zarit and B. G. Knight (Eds.), *A guide to psychotherapy and aging: Effective clinical interventions in a life-stage context* (pp. 61–82). Washington, D.C.: American Psychological Association.

Gallo, J. J., Rabins, P. V., Lyketsos, C. G., Tien, A. Y., and Anthony, J. C. (1997). Depression without sadness: Functional outcomes of nondysphoric depression in later life. *Journal of the American Geriatrics Society,* 45, 570–578.

Gatz, M., Johansson, B., Pedersen, N., Berg, S., and Reynolds, C. (1993). A cross-national self-report measure of depressive symptomatology. *International Psychogeriatrics,* 5, 147–156.

George, L. K. (1994). Social factors and depression in late life. In L. S. Schneider, C. F. Reynolds III, B. D. Lebowitz, and A. J. Friedhoff (Eds.), *Diagnosis and treatment of depression in late life: Results of the NIH Consensus Development Conference* (pp. 131–153). Washington, D.C.: American Psychiatric Press.

Gieselmann, B., and Bauer, M. (2000). Subthreshold depression in the elderly: Qualitative or quantitative distinction? *Comprehensive Psychiatry,* 41, 32–38.

Glasser, M., and Gravdal, J. A. (1997). Assessment and treatment of geriatric depression in primary care settings. *Archives of Family Medicine,* 6, 433–438.

Gloth, F. M., III. (2000). Geriatric pain: Factors that limit pain relief and increase complications. *Geriatrics,* 55, 46–48.

Grace, J., Nadler, J. D., White, D. A., Guilmette, T. J., Giuliano, A. J., Monsch, A. U., and Snow, M. G. (1995). Folstein vs. modified Mini-Mental State Examination in geriatric stroke: Stability, validity, and screening utility. *Archives of Neurology,* 52, 477–484.

Gradman, T. J., Thompson, L. W., and Gallagher-Thompson, D. (1999). Personality disorders and treatment outcomes. In E. Rosowsky, R. C. Abrams, and R. A. Zweig (Eds.), *Personality disorders in older adults: Emerging issues in diagnosis and treatment* (pp. 69–94). Mahwah, NJ.: Lawrence Erlbaum Associates.

Grundy, C. T., Lunnen, K. M., Lambert, M. J., Ashton, J. E., and Tovey, D. R. (1994). The Hamilton Rating Scale for Depression: One scale or many? *Clinical Psychology: Science and Practice,* 1, 197–205.

Haley, W. E., and Mangum, W. P. (1999). Ethical issues in geriatric assessment. In P. A. Lichtenberg (Ed.), *Handbook of assessment in clinical gerontology* (pp. 606–626). New York: John Wiley & Sons.

Haley, W. E., Han, B., and Henderson, J. N. (1998). Aging and ethnicity: Issues for clinical practice. *Journal of Clinical Psychology in Medical Settings,* 5, 393–409.

Hamilton, M. (1960). A rating scale for depression. *Journal of Neurology and Neurosurgical Psychiatry,* 23, 56–62.

Hartman-Stein, P. E. (Ed.). (1998). *Innovative behavioral healthcare for older adults: A guidebook for changing times.* San Francisco: Jossey-Bass Publishers.

Heckhausen, J., and Schulz, R. (1993). Optimisation by selection and compensation: Balancing primary and secondary control in life span development. *International Journal of Behavioral Development,* 16, 287–303.

Hegel, M. T., Barrett, J. E., and Oxman, T. E. (2000). Training therapists in problem-solving therapy of depressive disorders in primary care: Lessons learned from the "Treatment Effectiveness Project." *Family, Systems, and Health,* 18, 423–436.

Hillman, J. L. (2000). *Clinical perspectives on elderly sexuality.* New York: Kluwer Academic/Plenum Publishers.

Hinrichsen, G. A. (1999). Interpersonal psychotherapy for late-life depression. In M. Duffy (Ed.), *Handbook of counseling and psychotherapy with older adults* (pp. 470–486). New York: John Wiley & Sons.

Hinrichsen, G. A., and Zweig, R. (1994). Family issues in late-life depression. *Journal of Long-Term Home Health Care,* 13, 4–15.

Hoyl, M. T., Alessi, C. A., Harker, J. O., Josephson, K. R., Pietruszka, F. M., Koelfgen, M., Mervis, J. R., Fitten, L. J., and Rubenstein, L. Z. (1999). Development and testing of a five-item version of the Geriatric Depression Scale. *Journal of the American Geriatrics Society,* 47, 873–878.

Hunkeler, E. M., Meresman, J. F., Hargreaves, W. A., Fireman, B., Berman, W. H., Kirsch, A. J., Groebe, J., Hurt, S. W., Braden, P., Getzell, M., Feigenbaum, P. A., Peng, T., and Salzer, M. (2000). Efficacy of nurse telehealth care and peer support in augmenting treatment of depression in primary care. *Archives of Family Medicine, 9,* 700–708.

Hyer, L. (1999). The effects of trauma: Dynamics and treatment of PTSD in the elderly. In M. Duffy (Ed.), *Handbook of counseling and psychotherapy with older adults* (pp. 539–560). New York: John Wiley & Sons.

Irwin, M., Artin, K. H., and Oxman, M. N. (1999). Screening for depression in the older adult: Criterion validity of the 10-item Center for Epidemiological Studies Depression Scale (CES-D). *Archives of Internal Medicine,* 159, 1701–1704.

Jeste, D. V., Alexopoulos, G. S., Bartels, S. J., Cummings, J. L., Gallo, J. J., Gottlieb, G. L., Halpain, M. C., Palmer, B. W., Patterson, T. L., Reynolds, C. F., III, and Lebowitz, B. D. (1999). Consensus statement on the upcoming crisis in geriatric mental health: Research agenda for the next 2 decades. *Archives of General Psychiatry,* 56, 848–853.

Johnson, J., Weissman, M. M., and Klerman, G. L. (1992). Service utilization and social morbidity associated with depressive symptoms in the community. *Journal of the American Medical Association,* 267, 1478–1483.

Judd, L. L., Paulus, M. P., Wells, K. B., and Rapaport, M. H. (1996). Socioeconomic burden of subsyndromal depressive symptoms and major depression in a sample of the general population. *American Journal of Psychiatry,* 153, 1411–1417.

Kabacoff, R. I., Segal, D. L., Hersen, M., and Van Hasselt, V. B. (1997). Psychometric properties and diagnostic utility of the Beck Anxiety Inventory and the State-Trait Anxiety Inventory with older adult psychiatric outpatients. *Journal of Anxiety Disorders,* 11, 33–47.

Kalayam, B., and Alexopoulos, G. S. (1999). Prefrontal dysfunction and treatment response in geriatric depression. *Archives of General Psychiatry,* 56, 713–718.

Kaplan, M. S., Adamek, M. E., and Rhoades, J. A. (1998). Prevention of elderly suicide: Physicians' assessment of firearm availability. *American Journal of Preventive Medicine,* 15, 60–64.

Kaplan, M. S., Adamek, M. E., and Calderon, A. (1999). Managing depressed and suicidal geriatric patients: Differences among primary care physicians. *The Gerontologist,* 39, 417–425.

Karel, M. J. (1997). Aging and depression: Vulnerability and stress across adulthood. *Clinical Psychology Review,* 17, 847–879.

Karel, M. J. (2000). The assessment of values in medical decision making. *Journal of Aging Studies,* 14, 403–422.

Karel, M. J., and Hinrichsen, G. (2000). Treatment of depression in late life: Psychotherapeutic interventions. *Clinical Psychology Review,* 20, 707–729.

Katon, W., Robinson, P., Von Korff, M., Lin, E., Bush, T., Ludman, E., Simon, G., and Walker, E. (1996). A multifaceted intervention to improve treatment of depression in primary care. *Archives of General Psychiatry,* 53, 924–932.

Katon, W., Von Korff, M., Lin, E., Simon, G., Walker, E., Bush, T., and Ludman, E. (1997). Collaborative management to achieve depression treatment guidelines. *Journal of Clinical Psychiatry,* 58(Suppl. 1), 20–23.

Katon, W., Von Korff, M., Lin, E., Simon, G., Walker, E., Unützer, J., Bush, T., Russo, J., and Ludman, E. (1999). Stepped collaborative care for primary care patients with persistent symptoms of depression. *Archives of General Psychiatry,* 56, 1109–1115.

Katz, I. R. (1996). On the inseparability of mental and physical health in aged persons: Lessons from depression and medical comorbidity. *American Journal of Geriatric Psychiatry,* 4, 1–16.

Katz, I., and Coyne, J. C. (2000). The public health model for mental health care for the elderly. *Journal of the American Medical Association,* 283, 2844.

Kelly, K. G., and Zisselman, M. (2000). Update on electroconvulsive therapy (ECT) in older adults. *Journal of the American Geriatrics Society,* 48, 560–566.

Kemp, B. G., Corgiat, M., and Gill, C. (1992). Effects of brief cognitive-behavioral group psychotherapy with older persons with and without disabling illness. *Behavioral, Health, and Aging,* 2, 21–28.

Kirby, M., Bruce, I., Coakley, D., and Lawlor, B. A. (1999). Dysthymia among the community-dwelling elderly. *International Journal of Geriatric Psychiatry,* 14, 440–445.

Klerman, G. L., Weissman, M. M., Rounsaville, B. J., and Chevron, E. S. (1984). Interpersonal psychotherapy of depression. New York: Basic Books.

Knight, B. G., and McCallum, T. J. (1998). Adapting psychotherapeutic practice for older clients: Implications of the contextual, cohort-based, maturity, specific challenge model. *Professional Psychology: Research and Practice,* 29, 15–22.

Koenig, H. G., and Blazer, D. G. (1996). Minor depression in late life. *American Journal of Geriatric Psychiatry,* 4(Suppl. 1), S14-S21.

Koenig, H. G., George, L. K., and Siegler, I. C. (1988). The use of religion and other emotion-regulating coping strategies among older adults. *The Gerontologist,* 28, 303–310.

Koenig, H. G., Meador, K. G., Goli, V., Shelp, F., Cohen, H. J., and Blazer, D. G. (1992). Self-rated depressive symptoms in medical inpatients: Age and racial differences. *International Journal of Psychiatry in Medicine,* 22, 11–31.

Koenig, H. G., Cohen, H. J., Blazer, D. G., Krishnan, K. R. R., and Sibert, T. E. (1993). Profile of depressive symptoms in younger and older medical inpatients with major depression. *Journal of the American Geriatrics Society,* 41, 1169–1176.

Kominski, G., Anderson, R., Bastani, R., Gould, R., Hackman, C., Huang, D., Jarvik, L., Maxwell, A., Moye, J., Olsen, E., Rohrbaugh, R., Rosansky, J., Taylor, S., and Van Stone, W. (2001). UPBEAT: The impact of a psychogeriatric evaluation in VA medical centers. *Medical Care,* 39, 500-512.

Lawton, M. P. (1971). The functional assessment of elderly people. *Journal of the American Geriatrics Society,* 19, 465–481.

Lawton, M. P., and Brody, E. M. (1969). Assessment of older people: Self maintaining and instrumental activities of daily living. *The Gerontologist,* 9, 179–186.

Lazarus, L. W. (1988). Self psychology: Its application to brief psychotherapy with the elderly. *Journal of Geriatric Psychiatry,* 21, 109–125.

Lebowitz, B. D., Pearson, J. L., Schneider, L. S., Reynolds, C. F., III, Alexopoulos, G. S., Bruce, M. L., Conwell, Y., Katz, I. R., Meyers, B. S., Morrison, M. F., Mossey, J., Niederehe, G., and Parmalee, P. (1997). Diagnosis and treatment of depression in late life: Consensus statement update. *Journal of the American Medical Association,* 278, 1186–1190.

Lenze, E. J., Mulsant, B. H., Shear, M. K., Schulberg, H. C., Dew, M. A., Begley, A. E., Pollock, B. G., and Reynolds, C. F., III. (2000). Comorbid anxiety disorders in depressed elderly patients. *American Journal of Psychiatry,* 157, 722–728.

Leszcz, M. (1990). Toward an integrated model of group psychotherapy with the elderly. *International Journal of Group Psychotherapy,* 40, 379–399.

Liang, J., Tran, T. V., Krause, N., and Markides, K. S. (1989). Generational differences in the structure of the CES-D scale in Mexican Americans. *Journal of Gerontology,* 44, S110-S120.

Loewenstein, D. A., and Mogosky, B. J. (1999). The functional assessment of the older adult patient. In P. A. Lichtenberg (Ed.), *Handbook of assessment in clinical gerontology* (pp. 529–554). New York: John Wiley & Sons.

Lynch, T. R., Johnson, C. S., Mendelson, T., Robins, C. J., Krishnan, K. R. R., and Blazer, D. G. (1999). Correlates of suicidal ideation among an elderly depressed sample. *Journal of Affective Disorders,* 56, 9–15.

Lyness, J. M., Noel, T. K., Cox, C., King, D. A., Conwell, Y., and Caine, E. D. (1997). Screening for depression in elderly primary care patients. *Archives of Internal Medicine,* 157, 449–454.

MacNeill, S. E., and Lichtenberg, P. A. (1999). Screening instruments and brief batteries for assessment of dementia. In P. A. Lichtenberg (Ed.), *Handbook of assessment in clinical gerontology* (pp. 417–441). New York: John Wiley & Sons.

McCallum, J., Mackinnon, A., Simons, L., and Simons, J. (1995). Measurement properties of the Center for Epidemiological Studies Depression Scale: An Australian community study of aged persons. *Journal of Gerontology,* 50B, S182-S189.

McCusker, J., Cole, M., Keller, E., Bellavance, F., and Berard, A. (1998). Effectiveness of treatments of depression in older ambulatory patients. *Archives of Internal Medicine,* 158, 705–712.

McIntosh, J. L., Santos, J. F., Hubbard, R. W., and Overholser, J. C. (1994). *Elder suicide: Research, theory, and treatment.* Washington, D.C.: American Psychological Association.

Meeks, S. (1999). Bipolar disorder in the latter half of life: Symptom presentation, global functioning and age of onset. *Journal of Affective Disorders,* 52, 161–167.

Meyers, B. S., and Greenberg, R. (1986). Late-life delusional depression. *Journal of Affective Disorders,* 11, 133–137.

Miller, M. D., Frank, E., Cornes, C., Imber, S. D., Anderson, B., Ehrenpreis, L., Malloy, J., Silberman, R., Wolfson, L., Zaltman, J., and Reynolds, C. F. (1994). Applying interpersonal psychotherapy to bereavement-related depression following loss of a spouse in late life. *Journal of Psychotherapy Practice and Research,* 3, 149–162.

Morales, P. (1999). The impact of cultural differences in psychotherapy with older clients: Sensitive issues and strategies. In M. Duffy (Ed.), *Handbook of counseling and psychotherapy with older adults* (pp. 132–153). New York: John Wiley & Sons.

Morin, C. M., Landreville, P., Colecchi, C., McDonald, K., Stone, J., and Ling, W. (1999). The Beck Anxiety Inventory: Psychometric properties with older adults. *Journal of Clinical Geropsychology,* 5, 19–29.

Moye, J. (1999). Assessment of competency and decision making capacity. In P. A. Lichtenberg (Ed.), *Handbook of assessment in clinical gerontology* (pp. 488–528). New York: John Wiley & Sons.

Moye, J., Rosansky, J., Llorente, M., Jarvik, L., and the UPBEAT Collaborative Group. (2001). Engaging patients in treatment: Lesson learned from the UPBEAT Program. *Annals of Long-Term Care,* 9, 61–67.

Muldovsky, H., and Scarisbrick, P. (1976). Induction of neurasthenic musculoskeletal pain syndrome by selective sleep stage deprivation. *Psychosomatic Medicine,* 38, 35–44.

Mungas, D., Marshall, S. C., Weldon, M., Haan, M., and Reed, B. R. (1996). Age and education correction of Mini-Mental State Examination for English and Spanish-speaking elderly. *Neurology,* 46, 700–706.

Murrell, S. A., Himmelfarb, S., and Wright, K. (1983). Prevalence of depression and its correlates in older adults. *American Journal of Epidemiology,* 117, 173–185.

Mynors-Wallis, L. (1996). Problem-solving treatment: Evidence for effectiveness and feasibility in primary care. *International Journal of Psychiatry in Medicine,* 26, 249–262.

Nemiroff, R. A., and Colarusso, C. A. (Eds.). (1985). *The race against time: Psychotherapy and psychoanalysis in the second half of life.* New York: Plenum Press.

Newmann, J. P., Klein, M. H., Jensen, J. E., and Essex, M. J. (1996). Depression symptom experiences among older women: A comparison of alternative measurement approaches. *Psychology and Aging,* 11, 112–126.

Ostbye, T., Steenhuis, R., Walton, R., and Cairney, J. (2000). Correlates of dysphoria in Canadian seniors: The Canadian study of Health and Aging. *Canadian Journal of Public Health,* 91, 313–317.

O'Sullivan, R. L., Fava, M., Agustin, C., Baer, L., and Rosenbaum, J. F. (1997). Sensitivity of the six-item Hamilton Depression Rating Scale. *Acta Psychiatrica Scandinavica,* 95, 379–384.

Parmalee, P. A., Katz, I. R., and Lawton, M. P. (1993). Anxiety and its association with depression among institutionalized elderly. *American Journal of Geriatric Psychiatry,* 1, 46–58.

Penninx, B. W. J. H., Geerlings, S. W., Deeg, D. J. H., van Eijk, J. T. M., van Tilburg, W., and Beekman, A. T. F. (1999). Minor and major depression and the risk of death in older persons. *Archives of General Psychiatry,* 56, 889–895.

Prigerson, H. G., Frank, E., Kasl, S. V., Reynolds, C. F., III, Anderson, B., Zumbenko, G. S., Houck, P. R., George, C. J., and Kupfer, D. J. (1995a). Complicated grief and bereavement-related depression as distinct disorders: Preliminary empirical validation in elderly bereaved spouses. *American Journal of Psychiatry,* 152, 22–30.

Prigerson, H. G., Maciejewski, P. K., Reynolds, C. F., III, Bierhals, A. J., Newsom, J. T., Fasiczka, A., Frank, E., Doman, J., and Miller, M. (1995b). Inventory of complicated grief: A scale to measure maladaptive symptoms of loss. *Psychiatry Research,* 59, 65–79.

Qualls, S. H. (1995). Marital therapy with later life couples. *Journal of Geriatric Psychiatry,* 28, 139–163.

Qualls, S. H. (1999). Realizing power in intergenerational family hierarchies: Family reorganization when older adults decline. In M. Duffy (Ed.), *Handbook of counseling and psychotherapy with older adults* (pp. 228–241). New York: John Wiley & Sons.

Rabins, P. V., Black, B. S., Roca, R., German, P., McGuire, M., Robbins, B., Rye, R., and Brant, L. (2000). Effectiveness of a nurse-based outreach program for identifying and treating psychiatric illness in the elderly. *Journal of the American Medical Association,* 283, 2802–2809.

Radloff, L. S. (1977). The CES-D scale: A self-report depression scale for research in the general population. *Applied Psychological Measurement,* 1, 385–401.

Radloff, L. S., and Teri, L. (1986). Use of the Center for Epidemiological Studies Depression Scale with older adults. *Clinical Gerontology,* 5, 119–136.

Ramsey, J. L., and Blieszner, R. (2000). Transcending a lifetime of losses: The importance of spirituality in old age. In J. H. Harvey and E. D. Miller (Eds.), *Loss and trauma: General and close relationship perspectives* (pp. 225–236). Philadelphia: Brinner-Routledge/Taylor & Francis Group.

Rapp, S. R., Smith, S. S., and Britt, M. (1990). Identifying comorbid depression in elderly medical patients: Use of the extracted Hamilton Depression Rating Scale. *Psychological Assessment,* 2, 243–247.

Raschko, R. (1985). Systems integration at the program level: Aging and mental health. *The Gerontologist,* 25, 460–463.

Resick, P. A., and Schnicke, M. K. (1993). *Cognitive processing for rape victims: A treatment manual.* Newbury Park, Calif.: Sage Publications.

Reynolds, C. F., III. (1997). Treatment of major depression in later life: A life cycle perspective. *Psychiatric Quarterly,* 68, 221–246.

Reynolds, C. F., and Kupfer, D. J. (1999). Depression and aging: A look to the future. *Psychiatric Services,* 50, 1167–1172.

Reynolds, C. F., III, and Lebowitz, B. D. (1999). What are the best treatments for depression in old age? *Harvard Mental Health Letter,* 15, 8.

Reynolds, C. F., III, Frank, E., Perel, J. M., Imber, S. D., Cornes, C., Miller, M. D., Mazumdar, S., Houck, P. R., Dew, M. A., Stack, J. A., Pollock, B. G., and Kupfer, D. J. (1999). Nortriptyline and interpersonal psychotherapy as maintenance therapies for recurrent major depression: A randomized controlled trial in patients older than 59 years. *Journal of the American Medical Association,* 281, 39–45.

Rosenzweig, A., Prigerson, H., Miller, M. D., and Reynolds, C. F., III. (1997). Bereavement and late-life depression: Grief and its complications in the elderly. *Annual Review of Medicine,* 48, 421–428.

Rosowsky, E. (1999). Couple therapy with long-married older adults. In M. Duffy (Ed.), *Handbook of counseling and psychotherapy with older adults* (pp. 242–266). New York: John Wiley & Sons.

Rosowsky, E., and Smyer, M. A. (1999). Personality disorders and the difficult nursing home resident. In E. Rosowsky, R. C. Abrams, and R. A. Zweig (Eds.), *Personality disorders in older adults: Emerging issues in diagnosis and treatment* (pp. 257–274). Mahway, N.J.: Lawrence Erlbaum Associates.

Rosowsky, E., Dougherty, L. M., Johnson, C. J., and Gurian, B. (1997). Personality as an indicator of "goodness of fit" between the elderly individual and the health service system. *Clinical Gerontologist,* 17, 41–53.

Sackeim, H. A. (1994). Use of electroconvulsive therapy in late life depression. In L. S. Schneider, C. F. Reynolds, B. D. Lebowitz, and A. J. Friedhoff (Eds.), *Diagnosis and treatment of depression in late life* (pp. 259–277). Washington, D.C.: American Psychiatric Association Press.

Salzman, C. (1997). Depressive disorders and other emotional issues in the elderly: Current issues. *International Clinical Psychopharmacology,* 12(Suppl. 7), S37–42.

Schulz, R., Beach, S. R., Ives, D. G., Martire, L. M., Ariyo, A. A., and Kop, W. J. (2000). Association between depression and mortality in older adults: The cardiovascular health study. *Archives of Internal Medicine,* 160, 1761–1768.

Scogin, F. (2000). *The first session with seniors: A step-by-step guide.* San Francisco: Jossey-Bass Publishers.

Scogin, F., and McElreath, L. (1994). Efficacy of psychosocial treatments for geriatric depression: A quantitative review. *Journal of Consulting and Clinical Psychology,* 57, 403–407.

Scudds, R. J., and Robertson, J. M. (1998). Empirical evidence of the association between the presence of musculoskeletal pain and physical disability in community-dwelling senior citizens. *Pain,* 75, 229–235.

Shapiro, A. M., Roberts, J. E., and Beck, J. G. (1999). Differentiating symptoms of anxiety and depression in older adults: Distinct cognitive and affective profiles? *Cognitive Therapy and Research,* 23, 53–74.

Sheikh, J. I., and Yesavage, H. A. (1986). Geriatric Depression Scale (GDS): Recent evidence and development of a shorter version. *Clinical Gerontologist,* 5, 165–173.

Silver, I. L., and Herrmann, N. (1991). History and mental status examination. In J. Sadavoy, L. Lazarus, and L. Jarvik (Eds.), *Comprehensive review of geriatric psychiatry.* Washington, D.C.: American Psychiatric Press.

Simon, G. E., Von Korff, M., and Barlow, W. (1995). Health care costs of primary care patients with recognized depression. *Archives of General Psychiatry,* 52, 850–856.

Simon, G. E., Von Korff, M., Rutter, C., and Wagner, E. (2000). Randomized trial of monitoring, feedback, and management of care by telephone to improve treatment of depression in primary care. *British Medical Journal,* 320, 550–554.

Small, G. W., Rabins, P. V., Barry, P. P., Buckholtz, N. S., DeKosky, S. T., Ferris, S. H., Finkel, S. I., Gwyther, L. P., Khachaturian, Z. S., Lebowitz, B. D., McRae, T. D., Morris, J. C., Oakley, F., Schneider, L. S., Streim, J. E., Sunderland, T., Teri, L. A., and Tune, L. E. (1997). Diagnosis and treatment of Alzheimer disease and related disorders: Consensus statement of the American Association of Geriatric Psychiatry, the Alzheimer's Association, and the American Geriatrics Society. *Journal of the American Medical Association,* 278, 1363–1371.

Spitzer, R. L., Kroenke, K., Williams, J. B. W., and the Patient Health Questionnaire Primary Care Study Group. (1999). Validation and utility of a self-report version of PRIME-MD: The PHQ Primary Care Study. *Journal of the American Medical Association,* 282, 1737–1744.

Sprenkel, D. G. (1999). Therapeutic issues and strategies in group therapy with older men. In M. Duffy (Ed.), *Handbook of counseling and psychotherapy with older adults* (pp. 214–227). New York: John Wiley & Sons.

Steffens, D. C., Artigues, D. L., Ornstein, K. A., and Krishnan, K. R. R. (1997). A review of racial differences in geriatric depression: Implications for care and clinical research. *Journal of the National Medical Association,* 89, 731–736.

Stein, M. B., McQuaid, J. R., Pedrelli, P., Lenox, R., and McCahill, M. E. (2000). Posttraumatic stress disorder in the primary care medical setting. *General Hospital Psychiatry,* 22, 261–269.

Stiles, P. G., and McGarrahan, J. F. (1998). The Geriatric Depression Scale: A comprehensive review. *Journal of Clinical Geropsychology,* 4, 89–110.

Storandt, M., and VandenBos, G. R. (Eds.). (1995). *Neuropsychology assessment of dementia and depression in older adults: A clinician's guide.* Washington, D.C.: American Psychological Association.

Tait, R. C. (1999). Assessment of pain and response to treatment in older adults. In P. A. Lichtenberg (Ed.), *Handbook of assessment in clinical gerontology* (pp. 555–584). New York: John Wiley & Sons.

Teng, E. L., and Chui, H. C. (1987). The Modified Mini-Mental State (3MS) Examination. *Journal of Clinical Psychiatry,* 48, 314–318.

Teri, L., Truax, P., Logsdon, R., Uomoto, J., Zarit, S., and Vitaliano, P. P. (1992). Assessment of behavioral problems in dementia: The Revised Memory and Behavior Problems Checklist. *Psychology and Aging,* 7, 622–631.

Teri, L., Logsdon, R. G., Uomoto, J., and McCurry, S. M. (1997). Behavioral treatment of depression in dementia patients: A controlled clinical trial. *Journal of Gerontology,* 52B, P159-P166.

Thompson, L. W., Gallagher-Thompson, D., Futterman, A., Gilewski, M. J., and Peterson, J. (1991). The effects of late-life spousal bereavement over a thirty-month interval. *Psychology and Aging,* 6, 1–8.

Tobin, D. (1998). *Peaceful dying.* New York: Perseus Books.

Tombaugh, T. N., and McIntyre, N. J. (1992). The Mini-Mental State Examination: A comprehensive review. *Journal of the American Geriatrics Society,* 40, 922–935.

Tombaugh, T. N., McDowell, I., Kristjansson, B., and Hubley, A. M. (1996). Mini-Mental State Examination (MMSE) and the Modified MMSE (3MS): A psychometric comparison and normative data. *Psychological Assessment,* 8, 48–59.

Uncapher, H., and Arean, P. A. (2000). Physicians are less willing to treat suicidal ideation in older patients. *Journal of the American Geriatrics Society,* 48, 188–192.

Unützer, J., Patrick, D. L., Simon, G., Grembowski, D., Walker, E., Rutter, C., and Katon, W. (1997). Depressive symptoms and the cost of health services in HMO patients aged 65 years and older. *Journal of the American Medical Association,* 277, 1618–1623.

Unützer, J., Katon, W., Sullivan, M., and Miranda, J. (1999). Treating depressed older adults in primary care: Narrowing the gap between efficacy and effectiveness. *The Milbank Quarterly,* 77, 225–256.

Unützer, J., Simon, G., Belin, T. R., Datt, M., Katon, W., and Patrick, D. (2000). Care for depression in HMO patients aged 65 and older. *Journal of the American Geriatrics Society,* 48, 871–878.

Unützer, J., Katon, W. J., Williams, J. W., Callahan, C. M., Harpole, L., Hunkeler, E. M., Hoffing, M., Arean, P. A., Hegel, M. T., Schoenbaum, M., Oishi, S. M., and Langston, C. A. (2001). Improving primary care for depression in late life: The design of a multi-center randomized trial. *Medical Care,* 39, 785-799.

Weintraub, D., and Ruskin, P. E. (1999). Posttraumatic stress disorder in the elderly: A review. *Harvard Review of Psychiatry,* 7, 144–152.

Weissman, M. M., Bruce, M. L., Leaf, P. L., Florio, L. P., and Holzer, C., III. (1991). Affective disorders. In L. N. Robins and D. A. Regier (Eds.), *Psychiatric disorders in America: The Epidemiologic Catchment Area Study* (pp. 53–80). New York: The Free Press.

Weissman, M. M., Markowitz, J. C., and Klerman, G. L. (2000). *Comprehensive guide to interpersonal psychotherapy.* New York: Basic Books.

Wells, K. B., Stewart, A., Hays, R. D., Burnam, M. A., Rogers, W., Daniels, M., Berry, S., Greenfield, S., and Ware, J. (1989). The functioning and well-being of depressed patients: Results from the Medical Outcomes Study. *Journal of the American Medical Association,* 262, 914–919.

Wells, K. B., Sherbourne, C., Schoenbaum, M., Duan, N., Meredith, L., Unützer, J., Miranda, J., Carney, M. F., and Rubenstein, L. V. (2000). Impact of disseminating quality improvement programs for depression in managed primary care: A randomized controlled trial. *Journal of the American Medical Association,* 283, 212–220.

Wetherell, J. L., and Arean, P. A. (1997). Psychometric properties of the Beck Anxiety Inventory with older medical patients. *Psychological Assessment,* 9, 136–144.

Williams, J. B. W. (1988). A structured interview guide for the Hamilton Depression Rating Scale. *Archives of General Psychiatry,* 45, 742–747.

Williams, J. W., Barrett, J., Oxman, T., Frank, E., Katon, W., Sullivan, M., Cornell, J., and Sengupta, A. (2000). Treatment of dysthymia and minor depression in primary care: A randomized controlled trial in older adults. *Journal of the American Medical Association,* 284, 1519–1526.

Yale, R. (1995). *Developing support groups for individuals with early-stage Alzheimer's disease.* Baltimore: Health Professions Press.

Yesavage, J. A., Brink, T. L., Rose, T. L., Lum, O., Huang, V., Adey, M., and Leirer, V. O. (1983). Development and validation of a geriatric depression screening scale: A preliminary report. *Journal of Psychiatry Research,* 17, 37–49.

Young, R. C., and Klerman, G. L. (1992). Mania in late life: Focus on age at onset. *American Journal of Psychiatry,* 149, 867–876.

Zarit, S. H. (1996). Interventions with family caregivers. In S. H. Zarit and B. G. Knight (Eds.), *A guide to psychotherapy and aging: Effective clinical interventions in a life-stage context* (pp. 139–159). Washington, D.C.: American Psychological Association.

Zeiss, A. M., and Steffen, A. (1996). Behavioral and cognitive-behavioral treatments: An overview of social learning. In S. H. Zarit and B. G. Knight (Eds.), *A guide to psychotherapy and aging: Effective clinical interventions in a life-stage context* (pp. 35–60). Washington, D.C.: American Psychological Association.

Zeiss, A. M., and Zeiss, R. A. (1999). Sexual dysfunction: Using an interdisciplinary team to combine cognitive-behavioral and medical approaches. In M. Duffy (Ed.), *Handbook of counseling and psychotherapy with older adults* (pp. 294–313). New York: John Wiley & Sons.

Zeiss, A. M., Zeiss, R. A., and Davies, H. (1999). Assessment of sexual function and dysfunction in older adults. In P. A. Lichtenberg (Ed.), *Handbook of assessment in clinical gerontology* (pp. 270–296). New York: John Wiley & Sons.

Zweig, R. A., and Hillman, J. (1999). Personality disorders in adults: A review. In R. Rosowsky, R. C. Abrams, and R. A. Zweig (Eds.), *Personality disorders in older adults: Emerging issues in diagnosis and treatment* (pp. 31–53). Mahway, N.J.: Lawrence Erlbaum Associates.

Index

About the Authors

Michele J. Karel, Ph.D., is a practitioner, clinical supervisor, and researcher in geropsychology at the VA Boston Healthcare System and an Instructor in Psychology at Harvard Medical School. She lives in Waltham, Massachusetts.

Suzann M. Ogland-Hand, Ph.D., is a geriatric consultant and supervising geropsychologist with Pine Rest Christian Mental Health Services in Grand Rapids, Michigan, and an Adjunct Assistant Professor in the Department of Psychiatry at Michigan State University. She lives in Grand Rapids, Michigan.

Margaret Gatz, Ph.D., is Professor of Psychology at the University of Southern California. A leading academic in the field of geriatric mental health, she edited *Emerging Issues in Mental Health and Aging* (1995) after the last White House Conference on Aging and has authored more than 100 articles and book chapters. She lives in Los Angeles.

www.ingramcontent.com/pod-product-compliance
Ingram Content Group UK Ltd.
Pitfield, Milton Keynes, MK11 3LW, UK
UKHW021510180625
459791UK00013B/78/J

9 780465 095438